The Great Corn Odyssey

The History & Health Benefits of Corn

Joe Urbach

www.gardeningaustin.com

www.phytonutrientfarms.com

A

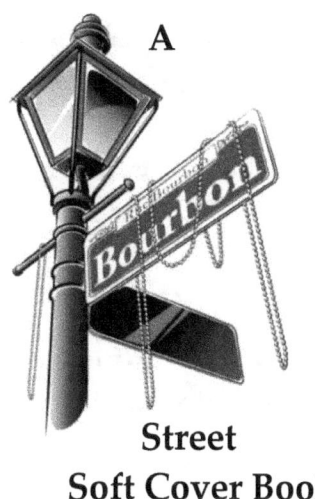

Street
Soft Cover Book

1st published in the United State in 2017 by
Bond Street Publications, a Hojo Enterprises Company

1st Printing 2017

DEDICATION

For Michael J.
An old friend who could eat corn by the bushel!

No waste either, the cobs were stripped bare
when he finished with them!

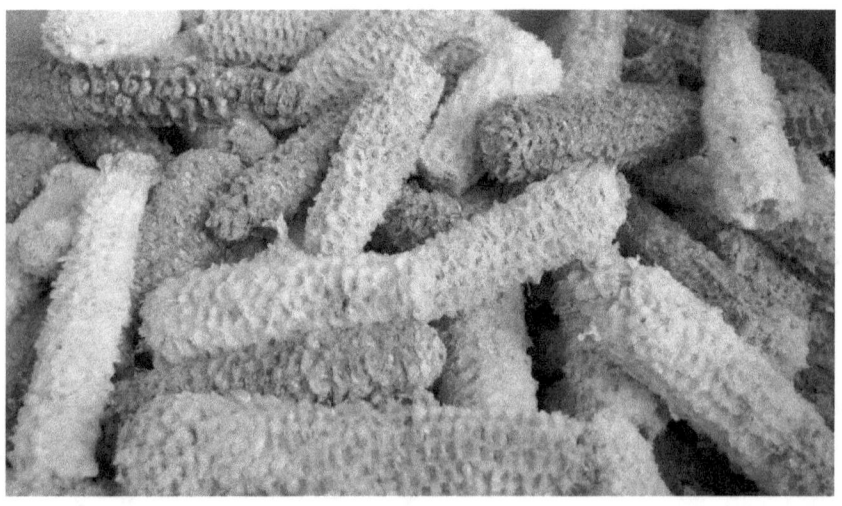

Corn Facts

Corn subsidies in the United States totaled $81.7 billion from 1995-2011. Corn draws in more subsidies than wheat, soybeans and rice combined

Americans consume one-third of all corn produced in the world.

It takes 91 gallons of water to produce one pound of corn. Annually, the industry uses 3.5 Long Island Sounds to grow crops.

Average corn yields have increased 500 percent since 1931, to 147.2 bu/acre from 24.5 bu/acre

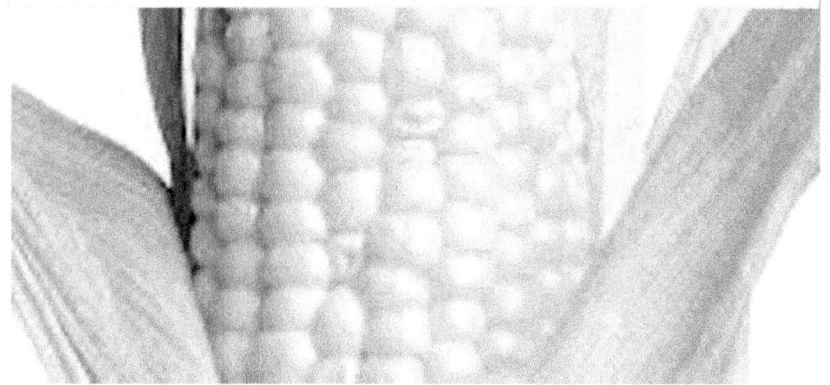

CONTENTS

Forward

   I am not a scientist, nor a medical doctor, nor a nutritionist nor any other kind of healthcare worker. If you have read any of my other books this will not be new information for you. I am not a research professional nor have I ever been involved in medical research of any kind.

I am a gardener, a father, a grandfather, and a diabetic. All of this led me to my concern about nutrition, and in turn, led me on a quest that eventually led to the writing of my _Yes, Food IS Medicine_ series of books, (originally titled 'Phytonutrient Gardening'). In which I present the 21st century science that proves to us that the food we eat, how we eat it, how we prepare it, how we store it, and even how we grow it, has a major impact on our health. My journey of exploration has convinced me that There really is a serious **PROBLEM** *with the* **NUTRITION-LESS** *state* of the modern fruits and vegetables that are finding their way into our local markets and then on to our very dinner plates. The real concern is that it soon can impact our health. In addition, half of the children on planet Earth live in terrible and, yes, inexcusable, poverty conditions, many suffering malnutrition and forced to drink polluted or tainted water. In this day and age, with all the modern advances of man, this situation is completely unacceptable and that was one driving force behind why I had to write that series.

   So, like many of you, I set off in search of helpful health information. Along the way, I learned some very useful and amazing things. I also uncovered some really fun and intriguing stories associated with the history of some of our favorite foods – but alas, most of what I found was of little merit and even less use. I found misinformation, false information, and outright lies. Much of the worst of the 'garbage' info I found revolved around many of my favorite foods and beverages such as, coffee, chocolate, alcohol, potatoes, corn, and so forth. I knew that someone was going to have to set the record straight; so, why not me!

The information I present in this work is provided for your consideration only and I absolutely do not condone, endorse, or recommend that you suddenly take up eating or drinking copious amounts of the food and drinks I will talk about here, in some crazy, misguided attempt to find a quick and easy health fix. *No. I do not even suggest you change any of your diet or exercise habits without first consulting your healthcare professional.*

My honest belief is that knowledge is power and my goal is to empower you with the information that follows so that you and your doctor can choose the best course of action for you to take to help you achieve a better, healthier, happier, more enjoyable, and longer life!

I Am Not A Doctor

The information presented here is accurate to the best of my knowledge.

I am not a doctor therefore this information is not intended to diagnose, treat, cure or prevent any disease because only doctors can do that.

Please do your own research!

INTRODUCTION

Over five hundred and twenty years ago, on a ship much like that pictured below, Christopher Columbus set sail in an attempt to find a new route to India. Instead he introduced Europe to the New World (notice I did not say that he discovered America – but more on that in a bit). Then on November 5, 1492, two of Columbus's men reported back to their captain from a journey to explore the interior of Cuba. Columbus recorded in his journal that the men had found the land planted with,

> *"a sort of grain they call Maize, which is very well tasted when boiled, roasted, or made into porridge."*

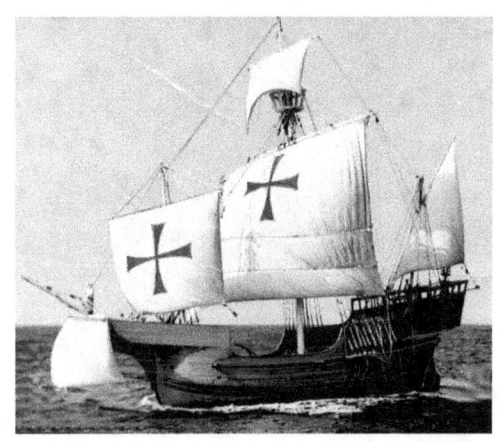

The story of corn and the early Americas is well-known. We know that the corn John Smith and Jamestown colonists stole from Indian caches helped them to stave off hunger; we know that the Whiskey Rebels cared about liquor less for drinking than as a way to get their fragile corn crop to distant markets. We know that the Ohio Valley, with its corn and hogs and whiskey, was a buffer between the North and South in the antebellum years, and how westward migration undercut the Ohio Valley Region's political power until it could no longer stave off war. But few of us pay much attention to the ancient or later history of corn, although there is no food in America that has a bigger effect on our lives. And there is no other food so truly American as corn. It is the country's biggest crop. Its origin is in the Americas. It is more

9

American than apple pie! Its history is both interesting and telling of how we human beings have been modifying our food for some 10,000 years! That's why I wrote this book, to share this festinating information and to, hopefully, teach as many people as possible how to grow, purchase, and consume the healthiest most phytonutrient-rich and antioxidant-dense corn we possibly can!

The USDA reported that in 2015, the nation produced a record corn crop of over 13.2 billion bushels. Only China comes close to the U.S. production of corn, but its production has not kept up with its growing population, and it has 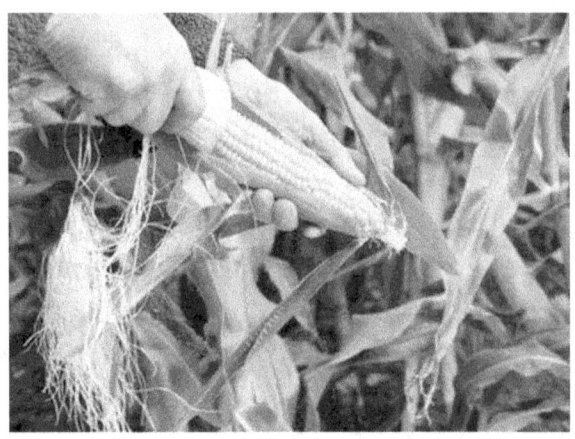 been importing US corn (at least until a few years back, when it rejected a US cargo ship full of corn because the ship contained a strain of genetically modified corn outside of trade agreements.)

The bright yellow, mouth-watering summer treat we all know so well does not grow in the wild _**anywhere**_ on planet Earth, so its ancestry was a mystery only recently discovered. While other grains such as oats, wheat and rice have obvious wild relatives, there is no wild plant that looks like our modern corn, with soft, starchy kernels arranged along a cob. None. Not anywhere on the planet. The abrupt appearance of corn in the archaeological record baffled scientists for many years. Some scientists concluded that the plant we know today arose through the domestication by early farmers and gardeners of a wild plant that was now extinct, or at least undiscovered. But with the help of modern science and some interesting lab work, that mystery has now been solved.

Good old corn on the cob, no other food has changed so dramatically from its ancient roots. Taking a quick look at corn's great odyssey is a good way of understanding how much our food has changed over the past 400 generations.

Corn, more properly called maize, is authentically American. The word "corn" comes from the Old English via Old Norse korn, meaning "grain." In most of the world, "corn" simply means the cereal crop most dominant in a region and can refer to any number of grains such as rye, wheat or oats. In the United States, what is known as corn was first called Indian corn; the adjective was commonly dropped by the early 1800s. (Although if you search "Indian corn" on the Internet, you'll notice that today the term refers to those dried multicolored cobs hanging around at Thanksgiving.) In practically every country but the United States, corn is called maize, coming from the Spanish maiz via the Taino mahiz.

Corn is the ancient grain of the New World. It was first cultivated 9,000 years ago and is a member of the grass family. We now know that it was first domesticated from a wild grain all those thousands of years ago by Aztec and Mayan Indians in Mexico and Central America.

For most of human history, our ancestors relied entirely on hunting animals and gathering seeds, fruits, nuts, tubers and other plant parts for food. It was only about 10,000 years ago that human beings, in many parts of the world, began raising livestock and growing food through deliberate planting. One of the first was maize.

We know that the history of modern-day corn begins thousands of years ago at the very dawn of human agriculture. Ancient gardeners took the first steps in domesticating maize when they simply chose which kernels (seeds) to plant. These clever folks noticed that not all plants were the same. Some plants may have grown larger than others, or maybe some kernels tasted better or were easier to grind. The gardeners saved kernels from plants with the most desirable characteristics and planted them for the next season's harvest. Many modern gardeners still do this today. This process is known as selective breeding or artificial selection. No real attempt was being made to change maize, these ancient people just wanted to plant what they liked best, just as we still do today. But little by little changes did occur, unwittingly the more they selected for what they liked best about their corn crops such as sweetness or more kernels, the more the phytonutrient content diminished.

Phytonutrients, also called phytochemicals, are chemicals produced by plants. Plants use phytonutrients to stay healthy. For example, some phytonutrients protect plants from insect attacks, while others protect against radiation from UV rays. Phytonutrients can also provide significant benefits for humans who eat those plants. Phytonutrient-rich foods include colorful fruits and vegetables, legumes, nuts, tea, whole grains and many spices. They affect human health but are not considered nutrients that are essential for life, like carbohydrates, protein, fats, vitamins and minerals. More and more research is showing that it is the phytonutrients in our foods that have the greater impact on our health.

So, for many generations, crop after crop of corn was selected, planted, selected again, planted again and so forth, over and over again. As a result of this selective breeding, maize cobs became larger over time, with more rows of kernels, eventually taking on the form of modern corn. But despite its abundance and importance, the biological origin of maize was still a long-running mystery.

The history of the development of modern corn fits right in with the traditional view of how our food changed over time. Local groups of gardeners selected the seeds to plant by choosing for those characteristics that they preferred and that worked best in their particular environments. Over thousands and thousands of years, selective breeding generated the broad diversity of corn varieties that are still grown around the world today. Unfortunately, this selective breeding had the unknown effect of breeding much of the nutritional value right out of our foods.

This was a completely unexpected result. No one planned this, worse yet we did not even know it had happened until the dawn of the 21st century! As a result, we have a problem **- the nutrition-less state of modern fruits and vegetables!** We all want healthy, nutritiously dense food on our tables, in our grocery stores, and in our gardens. But, the ugly truth is that this is not what we modern Americans are getting!

That may sound a bit bizarre to some, but it is none the less true. Modern science has proven ***beyond a shadow of a doubt*** that the fruit and vegetables we consume today are not only less nutritious than what our ancestors ate but are in fact, ***FAR LESS NUTRITIOUS!!***

Let's talk about that and a whole lot more as it applies to corn …

Chapter 1: Corn, an Ancient Mystery

As I begin this work, it is the beginning of the growing season across the Corn Belt of the United States. Seeds that have just been sown will, with a bit of help from Mother Nature in the form of just the right mixture of sunshine and rain, be knee-high plants by the Fourth of July and tall stalks with ears ripe for picking by late August.

Corn is much more than just a celebrated summer picnic food, however. Civilization owes much to this plant, and to the early people who first cultivated it! Food and food history interests me and the history and health benefits of corn is 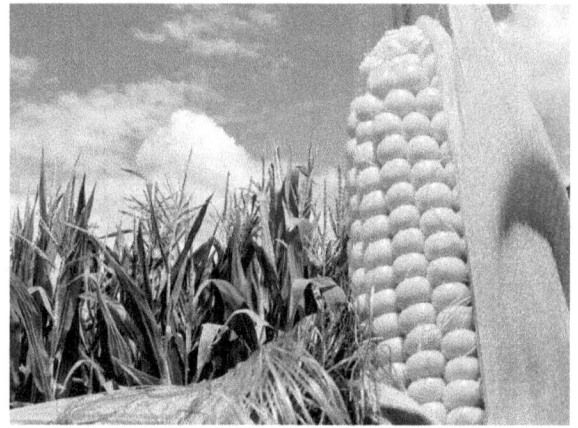 no exception. I hope you will find it as interesting as I do.

For most of human history, our ancestors relied entirely on hunting animals and gathering seeds, fruits, nuts, tubers and other plant parts from the wild for food. It was only about 10,000 years ago that humans in many parts of the world began raising livestock and growing food through deliberate planting. These advances provided more reliable sources of food and allowed for larger, more permanent settlements. Native Americans alone domesticated nine of the most important food crops in the world, including corn, more properly called maize (Zea mays to be exact), which now provides about 21 percent of human nutrition across the globe.

But despite its abundance and importance, the biological origin of maize had been a long-running mystery. The bright yellow, mouth-watering treat we know so well does not grow in the wild anywhere on planet Earth, so its ancestry was not at all obvious. That's right, corn as we know it today would not exist if it weren't for the humans that cultivated and developed it. It is a human invention, a plant that does not exist naturally in the wild. It can only survive if planted and protected by humans. Think about that, I find that to be extraordinarily intriguing.

Recently, however, the combined detective work of botanists, geneticists and archeologists has been able to identify the wild ancestor of maize, to pinpoint where the plant originated, and to determine when people were cultivating it and using it in their diets.

Enter a very clever Beadle.
The greatest surprise, and the source of much past controversy in corn archeology, was the identification of the ancient ancestor of maize. Many botanists did not see any connection between maize and other living plants. Some concluded that the crop plant arose through the domestication by early agriculturalists of a wild maize that was now extinct, or at least undiscovered.

However, one gifted scientist, working in the 1900s, uncovered evidence that linked maize to what, at first glance, would seem to be a very unlikely parent, a Mexican grass called teosinte. Looking at the skinny ears of teosinte, with just a dozen or so exposed kernels all wrapped inside a stone-hard casing, it is hard to see how they could be the forerunners of corn cobs with their many rows of juicy, naked kernels. Indeed, teosinte was at first classified as a grain closer to rice than to corn.

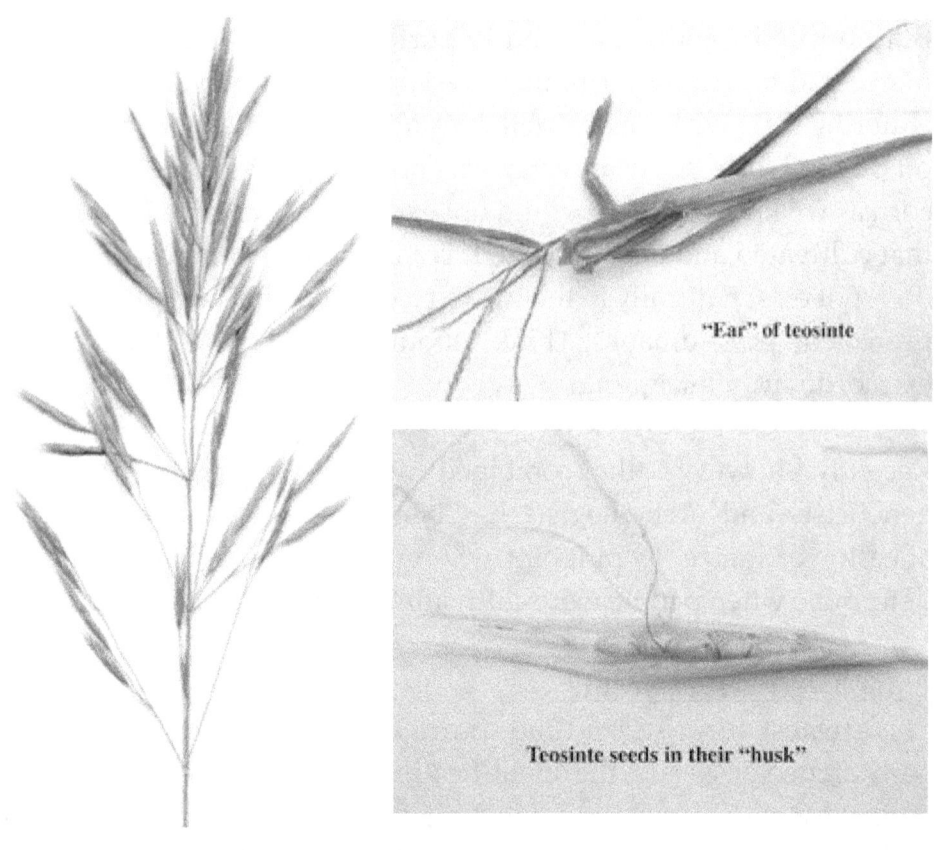

"Ear" of teosinte

Teosinte seeds in their "husk"

While a graduate student at Cornell University in the early 1930s, George W. Beadle found that maize and teosinte had very similar chromosomes. Moreover, he made fertile hybrids between maize and teosinte that looked like intermediates between the two plants. He even reported that he could get teosinte kernels to pop. Dr. Beadle concluded that the two plants were members of the same species, with maize being the domesticated form of teosinte. Dr. Beadle went on to make other, more fundamental discoveries in genetics for which he shared the Nobel Prize in 1958. He later became chancellor and president of the University of Chicago.

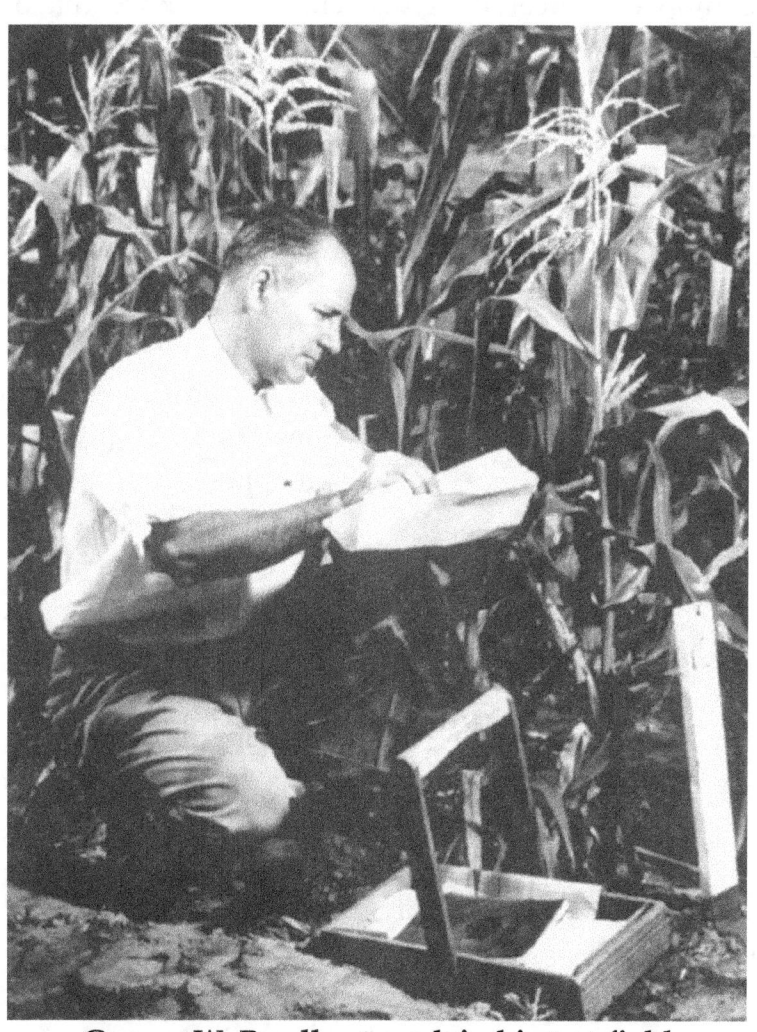

George W. Beadle at work in his test field.

Despite Dr. Beadle's illustrious reputation, his theory still remained in doubt three decades after he proposed it. The differences between the two plants appeared to many scientists to be too great to have evolved in just a few thousand years of domestication. So, after he formally retired, Dr. Beadle returned to the issue and sought ways to gather more evidence. As a great geneticist, he knew that one way to examine the parentage of two individuals was to cross them and then to cross their offspring and see how often the parental forms appeared. He crossed maize and teosinte, then crossed the hybrids, and **grew 50,000 plants.** He obtained plants that resembled teosinte and maize at a frequency that indicated that just four or five genes controlled the major differences between the two plants.

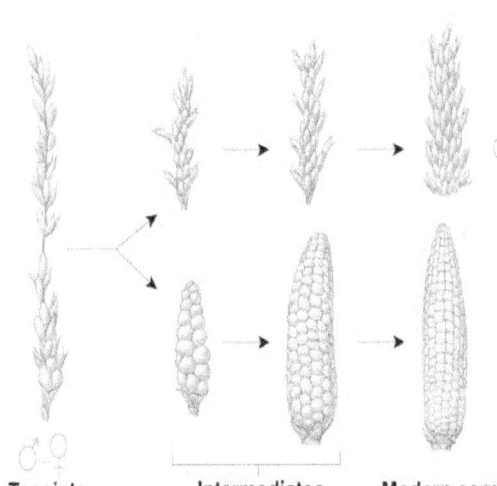

Teosinte   Intermediates   Modern corn

Dr. Beadle's results showed that maize and teosinte were without any doubt remarkably and closely related. But to pinpoint the geographic origins of maize, more definitive forensic techniques were needed. This was DNA typing, exactly the same technology used by the courts to determine paternity.

In order to trace maize's paternity, botanists led by John Doebley of the University of Wisconsin rounded up more than 60 samples of teosinte from across its entire geographic range in the Western Hemisphere and compared their DNA profile with all varieties of maize. They discovered that all maize was genetically most similar to a teosinte type from the tropical Central Balsas River Valley of southern Mexico, suggesting that this region was the "cradle" of maize evolution. Furthermore, by calculating the genetic distance between modern maize and Balsas teosinte, they estimated that domestication occurred about 9,000 years ago.

These genetic discoveries inspired recent archeological excavations of the Balsas region that sought evidence of maize use and to better understand the lifestyles of the people who were planting and harvesting it. Researchers led by Anthony Ranere of Temple University and Dolores Piperno of the Smithsonian National Museum of Natural History excavated caves and rock shelters in the region, searching for tools used by their inhabitants, maize starch grains and other microscopic evidence of maize.

In the Xihuatoxtla shelter, they discovered an array of stone milling tools with maize residue on them. The oldest tools were found in a layer of deposits that were 8,700 years old. This is the earliest physical evidence of maize use obtained to date, and it coincides very nicely with the time frame of maize domestication estimated from DNA analysis.

The most impressive aspect of the maize story is what it tells us about the capabilities of agriculturalists 9,000 years ago. These people were living in small groups and shifting their settlements seasonally. Yet they were able to transform a grass with many inconvenient, unwanted features into a high-yielding, easily harvested food crop. The domestication process must have occurred in many stages over a considerable length of time as many different, independent characteristics of the plant were modified.

The most crucial step was freeing the teosinte kernels from their stony cases. Another step was developing plants where the kernels remained intact on the cobs, unlike the teosinte ears, which shatter into individual kernels. Early cultivators had to notice among their stands of plants variants in which the nutritious kernels were at least partially exposed, or whose ears held together better, or that had more rows of kernels, and they had to selectively breed them. It is estimated that the initial domestication process that produced the basic maize form required at least several hundred to perhaps a few thousand years.

Using the modern techniques of today, another group of scientists analyzed the DNA from teosinte-maize offspring. Like Dr Beadle, the too noticed that about 5 regions of the genome (which could be single genes or could be groups of genes) seemed to be controlling the most significant differences between teosinte and maize.

I know that this may be a bit confusing so let me try to simplify it...

What all of this mumbo jumbo means is that the earliest events in maize domestication most likely involved **small** changes to **single genes** that in turn had **dramatic effects**. We know the events were early because there is little variation in these genes between maize varieties, suggesting that modern varieties are *descended from a single ancestor*. So, today we know that the history of modern-day maize did, in fact, begin at the dawn of human agriculture, about 10,000 years ago.

Ancient farmers in what is now Mexico took the first steps in domesticating maize

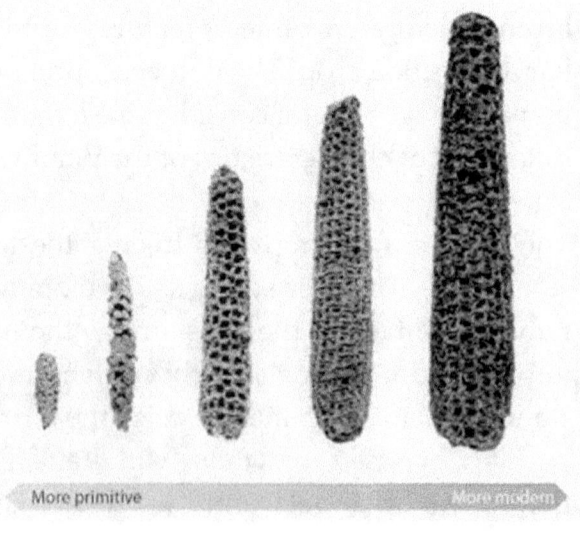

More primitive   More modern

when they simply chose which kernels (seeds) to plant. These farmers noticed that not all plants were the same. Some plants may have grown larger than others, or maybe some kernels tasted better or were easier to grind. The farmers saved kernels from plants with desirable characteristics and planted them for the next season's harvest. This process is known as selective breeding or artificial selection. Maize cobs became larger over time, with more rows of kernels, eventually taking on the form of modern maize.

The identity of maize's wild ancestor, while it had remained a mystery for many decades, was no known. While other grains such as wheat and rice have obvious wild relatives, there is no wild plant that looked like maize, with soft, starchy kernels arranged along a cob. The abrupt appearance of maize in the archaeological record had scientists baffled. Evolution was generally thought to occur gradually through minor changes. Why did maize appear so suddenly?

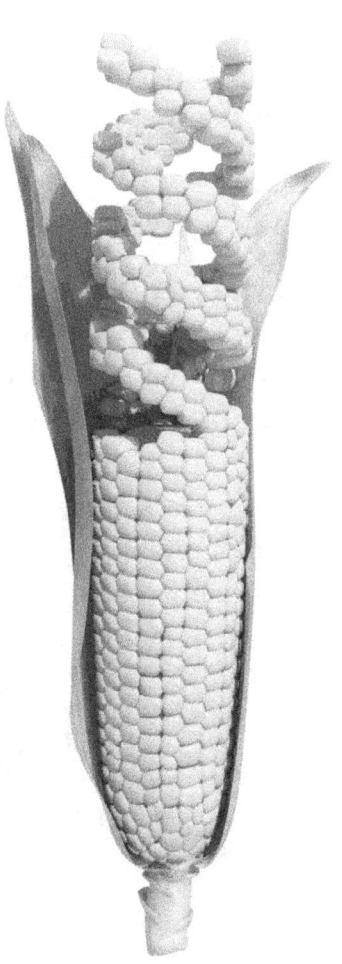

Thanks to modern science, through the study of genetics, we now know that corn's wild ancestor is actually a grass called teosinte. Teosinte doesn't look much like maize, especially when you compare its kernels to those of corn. But at the DNA level, the two are surprisingly alike. They have the same number of chromosomes and a remarkably similar arrangement of genes. In fact, teosinte can cross-breed with modern maize varieties to form maize-teosinte hybrids that can go on to reproduce naturally.

Scientists study teosinte-maize hybrids and their offspring through the process of genetic archaeology. This process helps geneticists understand what is happening at the DNA level to make teosinte and maize so different. By combining clues from genetics and the archaeological record, scientists have pieced together much of the story of maize evolution.

One of the first scientists to fully appreciate the close relationship between teosinte and maize was George W. Beadle. In the 1930s, Beadle studied teosinte-maize hybrids and showed that their chromosomes are highly compatible. Later, he produced large numbers of teosinte-corn hybrids and observed the characteristics of their offspring. By applying basic laws of genetic inheritance, Beadle calculated that only about 5 genes were responsible for the most-notable differences between teosinte and a primitive strain of maize.

In recent years, geneticists have used advanced molecular-biology tools to pinpoint the roles of some of the genes with large effects, as well as many other regions across the genome that have had subtle effects on maize domestication.

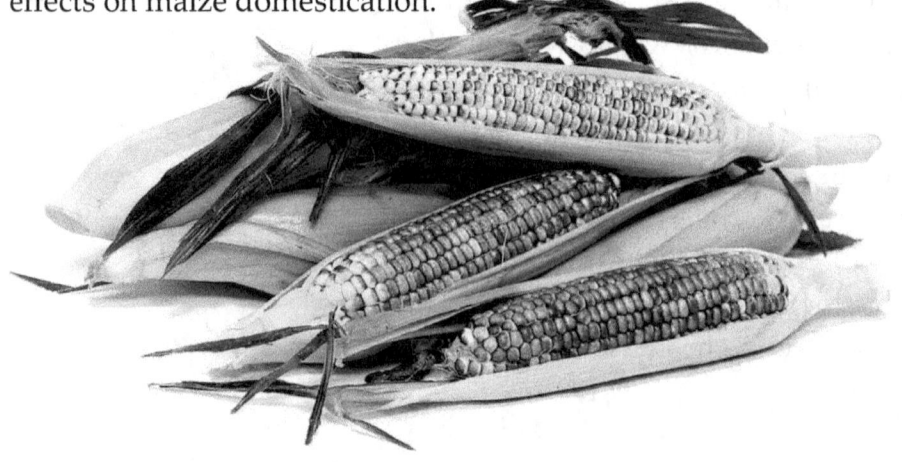

The earliest events in maize domestication likely involved small changes to single genes with dramatic effects. We know the events were early because there is little variation in these genes between maize varieties, suggesting that modern varieties are descended from a single ancestor. That the small changes had dramatic effects also explains the sudden appearance of maize in the archaeological record. These examples show us that evolution doesn't always involve gradual change over time.

Later changes in the evolution of modern maize involved many genes (perhaps thousands) with small effects. These minor changes include the following:

- Types and amounts of starch production
- Ability to grow in different climates and types of soil
- Length and number of kernel rows
- Kernel size, shape, and color
- Resistance to pests

These examples fit with the traditional view of evolution as gradual change over time. Local groups of farmers selected for characteristics that they preferred, and that worked best in their particular environment. Over thousands of years, selective breeding generated the broad diversity of corn varieties that are still grown around the world today.

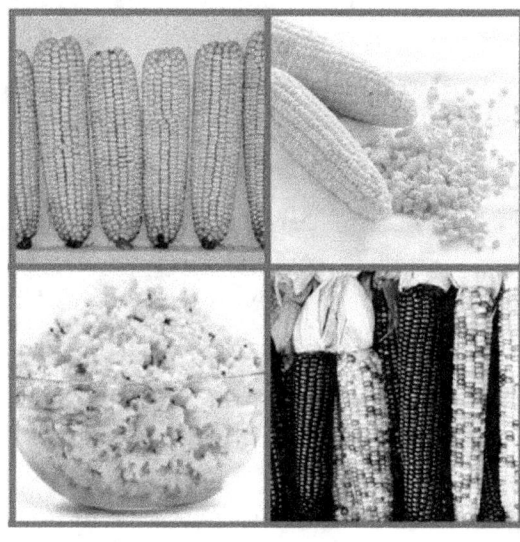

Chapter 2: Corn in Ancient America

If you could pick a single food that exemplifies the Americas, what would you pick? No food really screams American like corn (except perhaps the hotdog or hamburger). In the U.S., corn is popular in every state and really shows up in Southern food. Some popular corn dishes in the South include cornbread (also known as hoecakes or johnny cakes among Southerners), corn pudding, creamed corn, succotash, and old fashioned buttered corn on the cob.

It'll give you an idea of just how central corn has always been to the American diet when you consider a little bit of corn history...

Corn is completely native to the Americas. It was grown exclusively by the Native Americans, thousands of years before Christopher Columbus journeyed to the New World. Petrified cobs have been discovered that are thousands of years old to prove this. The Native American name for corn was mahiz, which the early settlers called maize. In Native American language usage, the word "mahiz" means "that which sustains us." "Corn" originally was an English term used to denote small particles, particular grains. Corned beef received it's moniker from the small grains (corns) of salt used to preserve it. What we now call corn the early American colonists called Indian corn which was eventually lexicalized to corn. Today, "Indian Corn" refers to the ornamental corn of Halloween and Thanksgiving fame.

Cultivating corn is responsible for turning the Native American tribes from nomadic to agrarian societies. They even used corn to brew beer before the European settlers arrived.

Mesoamerica is a region straddling the southern part of North America and the northern part of Central America. Long obscured by modern day political boundaries it roughly encompasses the southern half of Mexico and the north-western section of Central America. It was a cradle of Pre-Columbian (before Columbus) civilization and was home to the renowned Maya and Aztec Indians, amongst others. Sadly, as with the North American continent, the cultural richness of these peoples, not to mention their way of life, was all but destroyed by the European imperialists, in this particularly tragic case, the Spanish. But all the European might could not vanquish some of the timeless gifts these people left to mankind; one of the most amazing being maize, otherwise known as corn in the United States.

(Another of these gifts is chocolate – I wrote a book about chocolate too! It is called ***Wine, Chocolate, & your Good Health!*** You can find it at my website: www.gardeningaustin.com/store)

But the term "corn" is not the only aspect of this bountiful vegetable to be morphed over the ages. The plant itself is truly a bit of a transmutation. Although the exact seminal plant species was unknow until the 20th century, what you and I refer to as "corn" in the modern-day supermarket aisle, is not what first sprouted in the New World. The predecessor of today's corn began somewhere in the Andes. The Andean Indians introduced it to Central America where it eventually made its way to Mexico. There are an array of theories outlining the specific ontogenesis but basically, sometime between 10,000 and 5,500 BC the first corn plants appear to have become hybridized and domesticated. Sometime between 8,000 and 5,000 BC maize was flourishing in Mesoamerica. Archaeological evidence confirms at least 3,600 BC but it is inescapable that the process was in motion well before that.

Strangely, despite thousands of years of cultivation in the lower Americas, corn didn't find its way to the modern day United States (except for a small part of the most southern regions of New Mexico) until around about 1000 years ago. By 600 AD a number of North American Indians were extensively growing it. Corn's journey to the Old World began with Christopher Columbus who ferried it back to Spain. By 1500 AD it was under cultivation in Spain and by the 17th century it was a major crop for a number of European countries. The Portuguese introduced it to East Africa and Asia and from there it was just a matter of time until it arrived in India and China through established trade routes. It was flourishing in China in the 18th century and reached Korea and Japan soon after. Corn is now one of the most widely grown vegetables on Earth, especially in the Americas. The United States and China lead world production.

Remarkably, the early Spanish invaders of Mesoamerica were aversive to corn. Some of the Indian tribes practiced human sacrifice and grisly rituals which involved corn. The conquistadors thus correlated corn with destructive paganism and considered its consumption to be wholly unchristian. Corn consumption was also associated with pellagra, a deficiency disease of niacin in conjunction with the amino acid tryptophan. Corn is lacking in niacin. Tryptohan can be converted to niacin in the body thus decreasing the depletion of niacin. A diet dominated by corn with little other vegetables or sources of tryptophan can result in pellagra. Pellagra causes dermatological, gastrointestinal and neurological symptoms and ultimately death. Eventually of course, the Europeans out-grew their initial prejudices against corn.

What is truly amazing about corn is its versatility and seemingly innumerable uses. Not even considering the culinary uses, (which I'll address later), the list is impressive.

Morphology of Maize

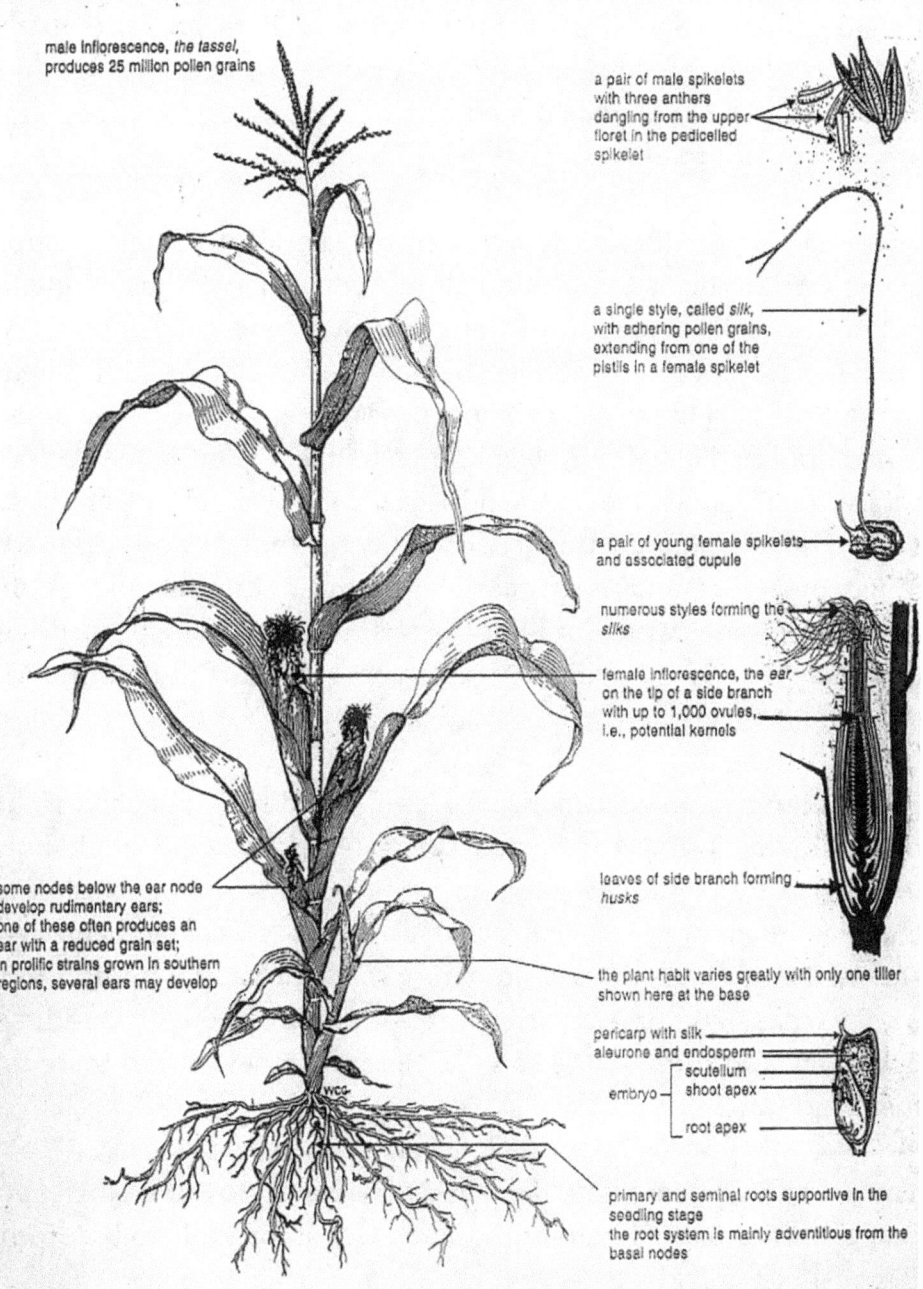

male inflorescence, *the tassel*, produces 25 million pollen grains

a pair of male spikelets with three anthers dangling from the upper floret in the pedicelled spikelet

a single style, called *silk*, with adhering pollen grains, extending from one of the pistils in a female spikelet

a pair of young female spikelets and associated cupule

numerous styles forming the *silks*

female inflorescence, the *ear* on the tip of a side branch with up to 1,000 ovules, i.e., potential kernels

some nodes below the ear node develop rudimentary ears; one of these often produces an ear with a reduced grain set; in prolific strains grown in southern regions, several ears may develop

leaves of side branch forming *husks*

the plant habit varies greatly with only one tiller shown here at the base

pericarp with silk
aleurone and endosperm
scutellum
embryo — shoot apex
root apex

primary and seminal roots supportive in the seedling stage
the root system is mainly adventitious from the basal nodes

The Indians wove the husks into clothing, sleeping mats, baskets, and children's toys. Most of the corn grown in the United States and Canada today is used as animal fodder. There are also many industrial uses of corn including ethanol, cosmetics, ink, glue, laundry starch, shoe polish, medicines, fabrics, corncob pipes, and ornaments, just to name a few.

There are many different types of corn. The most notable include Sweet Corn. This is the traditional favorite, eaten off the cob with butter and salt, and found in supermarkets and roadside stands everywhere. Sweet corn is so named because of its high sugar content. It is seldom used for purposes other than direct human consumption. Dent Corn, also known as Field Corn is the corn of choice for livestock feed and industrial products. Flint Corn, also known as the aforementioned ornamental Indian Corn sports a range of colors and is primarily grown in Central and South America. A sub variety of Flint Corn is used to make popcorn. Its soft starchy center facilitates the "pop" into the fluffy, movie-snacking favorite.

The earliest settlers in America may very well have perished if the natives hadn't introduced them to corn. The settlers were taught how to grow it by planting kernels in small holes with small fish and covering them up. The fish acted as fertilizer. The Indians also shared their various ways of preparing corn, such as pounding it into meal to make cornbread, corn soup, corn cakes, and corn pudding. Corn was also used by the early settlers as money and to trade for meat and furs.

The love of corn goes very deep and way back into our history. The first governor of the Plymouth Colony, Governor William Bradford, famously once said:

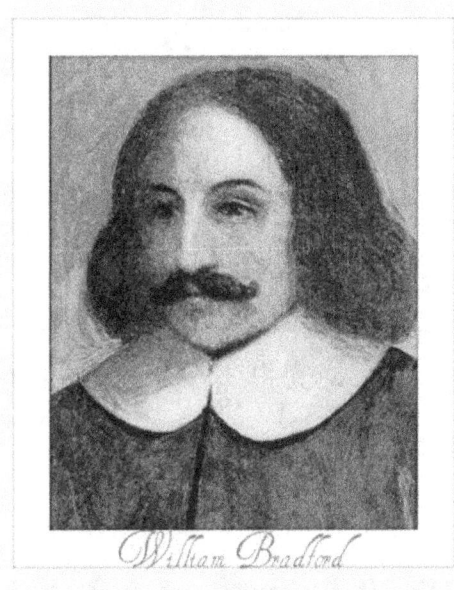

William Bradford

"And sure it was God's good providence that we found this corne for we know not how else we should have done."

And the reverence for corn that the settlers in the U.S. had back then still goes on today. It's the largest crop in the U.S. It regularly graces dinner tables, including Thanksgiving dinner ever since the year 1621. Small towns all around America's heartland celebrate the harvest with corn festivals. In Iowa, the nation's #1 corn producer, about half the farming land is devoted to just corn! In my part of Texas, the fields are planted 3 times every year, with cotton, sorghum and corn.

It's also one of the most widely distributed crops in the world. In fact, street vendors around the world sell husked corn, which developed from American settlers adapting the native style of roasting corn without the husks.

Chapter 3: Corn Proves the Point

Was Columbus the first to discover America or is it possible that there was pre-Columbian contact between the Old World and the New World? In general, scholars concerned with the ancient culture history of the Americas, believe that there were little or no significant connections by voyaging between the Old World and the New World before 1492.

The key word here is 'significant' as in…

"Sure, the Vikings found North America and maybe the Chinese found the Pacific Northwest but there was never any trade or other 'advanced or significant' contact between the Old World and the New World before Columbus' voyage in the 15ᵗʰ century."

Personally, I just do not buy it, and I can show you that corn (maize) proves it!

No significant contact between the Old World and the New World before 1492. What a load of hogwash! To the contrary, data from extensive literature that hitherto has been inadequately searched demonstrates that some fauna and flora, such as American Corn were extensively shared between the Old and New Worlds before Columbus' discovery of the Americas. The only plausible explanation for this bi-hemispheric distribution is that those shared organisms moved across the oceans via intentional voyages that took place during the eight millennia or more immediately preceding Columbus' so called, discoveries. This chapter presents and documents the evidence for this position. I really believe that students of the human past are obliged to adopt a new paradigm for the role of long-distance sea communication in history and in culture.

The literature on the question of whether maize (corn - Zea mays) appeared in Eurasia before the time of Columbus has become large and contentious. Few botanists and even fewer archaeologists or historians have combed that literature exhaustively. I cannot claim to have done so either, but I have read enough to know that a close look at corn tells the tale!

My research suggests that in the past, arguments for transoceanic contacts have relied mainly on evidence from cultural parallels and not from the evidence of flora and fauna. Some of those parallels are indeed striking, but scholars generally have rejected their value as evidence that significant pre-Columbian contacts took place with the Americas across the oceans. Over a century ago, one scholar named Tylor, in 1896 compared details of the Aztec board game, patolli eg, the board's layout, the sequence of moves, and cosmic associations of the pieces and moves, with the game called pachisi in India. Even Robert Lowie in 1951, an influential anthropologist who was usually critical of diffusionist (voyage-dependent) explanations for the occurrence of such similarities, accepted that in this case "the concatenation of details puts the parallels far outside any probability of having been invented independently." Still, tentative acceptance by some influential observers, like Lowie, of the possible historical significance of the cultural parallels has always ended up being rebutted by a demand from critics for 'hard,' or 'scientific' evidence for voyaging. Often, the sort of evidence demanded was demonstration that numbers of plants were present on both sides of the oceans before Columbus' day.

I do not believe that we must find evidence of *"numbers of plants present on both sides of the oceans before Columbus' day"* to prove this. I mean, think about it, if even a single plant that can only be propagated by man (such as corn) is found in Asia or Africa at any time before 1492, we must then recognize that 'significant' pre-Columbian contact did indeed exist between the Old World and the New world in the days before Columbus landed his ships in the Americas. Period.

Many recent field investigations have discovered odd sorts of maize growing in Asia (especially Sikkim Primitive in the remote Himalaya and 'waxy' varieties from Myanmar {Burma} all across China to the Korean peninsula), mostly away from coastal areas where 16th century Iberian sailors are supposed to have first introduced maize. The characteristics and distribution of these grains cannot be explained in terms of post-Columbian introduction, because waxy varieties were not known in the Americas at that time. Yet, some unusual traits exhibited in these Asian maizes have close matches to corn known archaeologically from Peru, or that is still being grown by native groups in Peru, Colombia, Chile, Bolivia, and Argentina.

Utterly decisive evidence for the presence of American maize in the Old World has been found in Asian art and archaeology. These were the first items to document extensively that corn ears were represented in sculptures in India — hundreds of them — on original temple walls in Karnataka State, southern India. This art absolutely dates from the 11th to the 13th centuries AD, but there are some representations that date to be very much older. This is clearly well before Columbus sailed the ocean blue in 1492.

Researches have now independently identified maize, as well as a number of other plants of American origin, sculpted on Indian temples and monuments. The evidence of maize in archaeological sites in China and its depiction in Hoysala Temples in India, both dated before the 15th century AD, suggests that this domesticated crop was diffused by human action before the arrival of Columbus in the New World. The implications of this evidence are of great magnitude, since the presence of maize in Asia indicates that humans were able to migrate between both hemispheres; more than likely through trans-oceanic means of travel.

So, let's see the evidence…

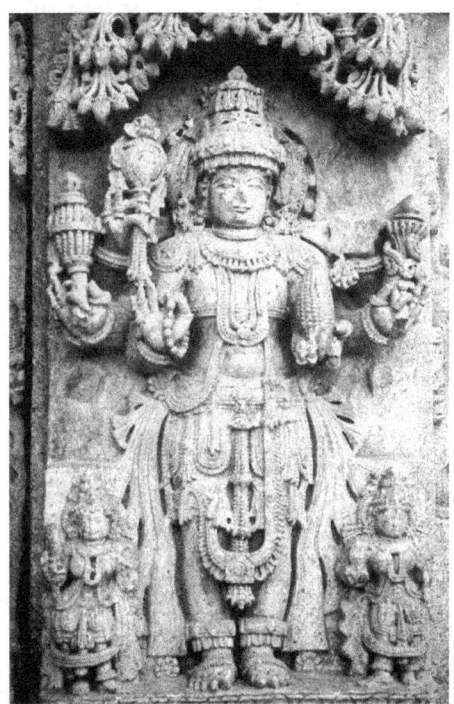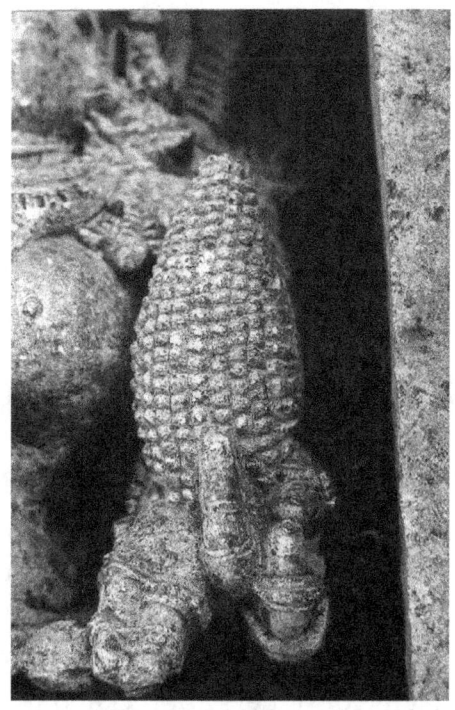

The above sculptures are built into temples as load bearing walls with mortise and tenon joints at top and bottom of each sculpted block. They bear the load of stone beams and stone roofs on top.

Temples are dated in written historical records in South India. They contain who built the structures, when they were built, the cause for which they were built, and who the sculptors were. Archaeological discoveries in the last decade have similar carvings of maize, etc., and indicate that the sculptural work was typical of sculptures of the reigning Hoysala Dynasty of the **11th to 13th centuries**. Yes, that is indeed several hundred years before Columbus was even born.

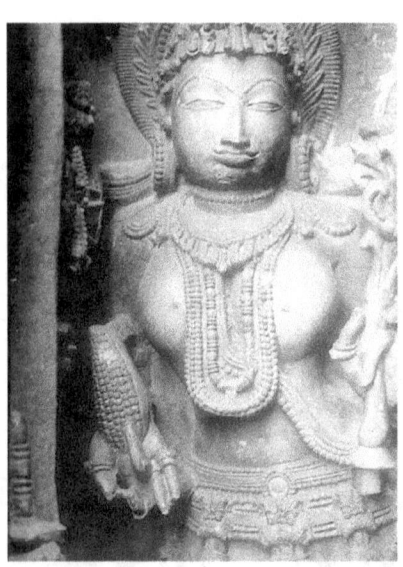 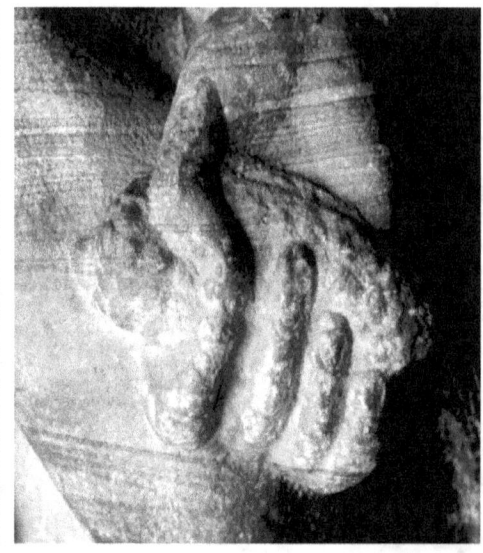

Direct observations in the temples show that no two maize ears are identical. Each of the more than 100 temples has similar carvings. Over 80 large ears are present in the last and most beautiful Somnathpur temple with several hundred examples of smaller ears elsewhere, in the roof for example, and these corn ears demonstrate that the designers appreciated the multi-seeded fertility symbol, just as they carved the images of the Annonas and sunflowers, which are multi-seeded fruits decorating the walls and courtyards.

Maize breeders in India, China, United States, and Great Britain, who have seen extensive collections of the illustrations, concur that only sculptors with abundant ears of maize as models could have created these illustrations of maize. No other biological product has these assemblages of anatomical characteristics that are within the envelope of variations of maize. I grant that these findings have been thought to be impossible in the earlier belief systems that maintained that there was no significant contact between New and Old World. These anti-diffusionist beliefs have to give way to reality.

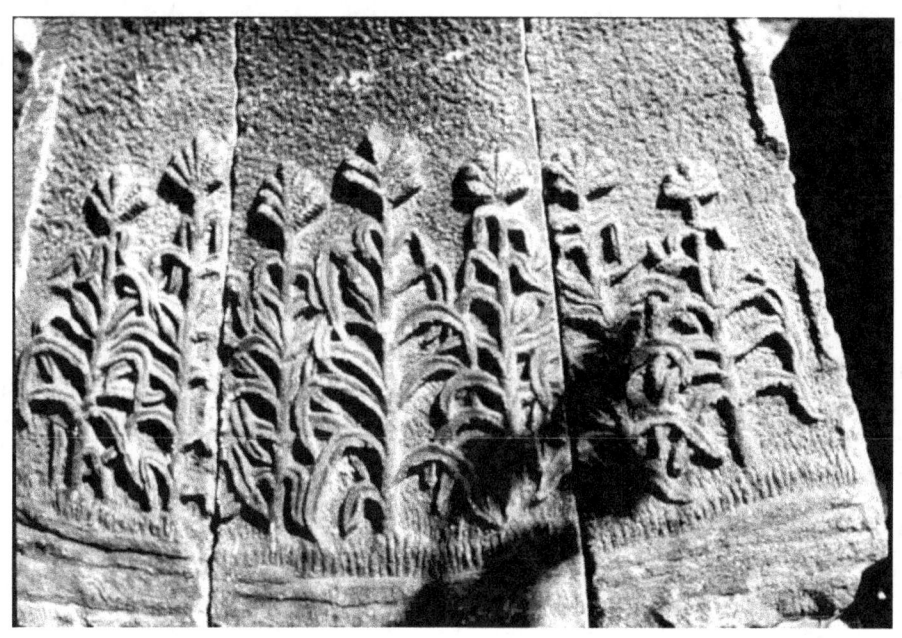

Archaeological findings have been found to verify this and archaeologists are currently finding much more evidence of contact between Asia and the Americas. Many of these relate to DNA complexity of biotic forms that can be tested for indications of genetic similarities and genetic distances, but written literature, paintings, sculptures, and archaeological finds all support not detract from the diffusion hypothesis of very ancient sailing contact in the building of high civilizations around the world.

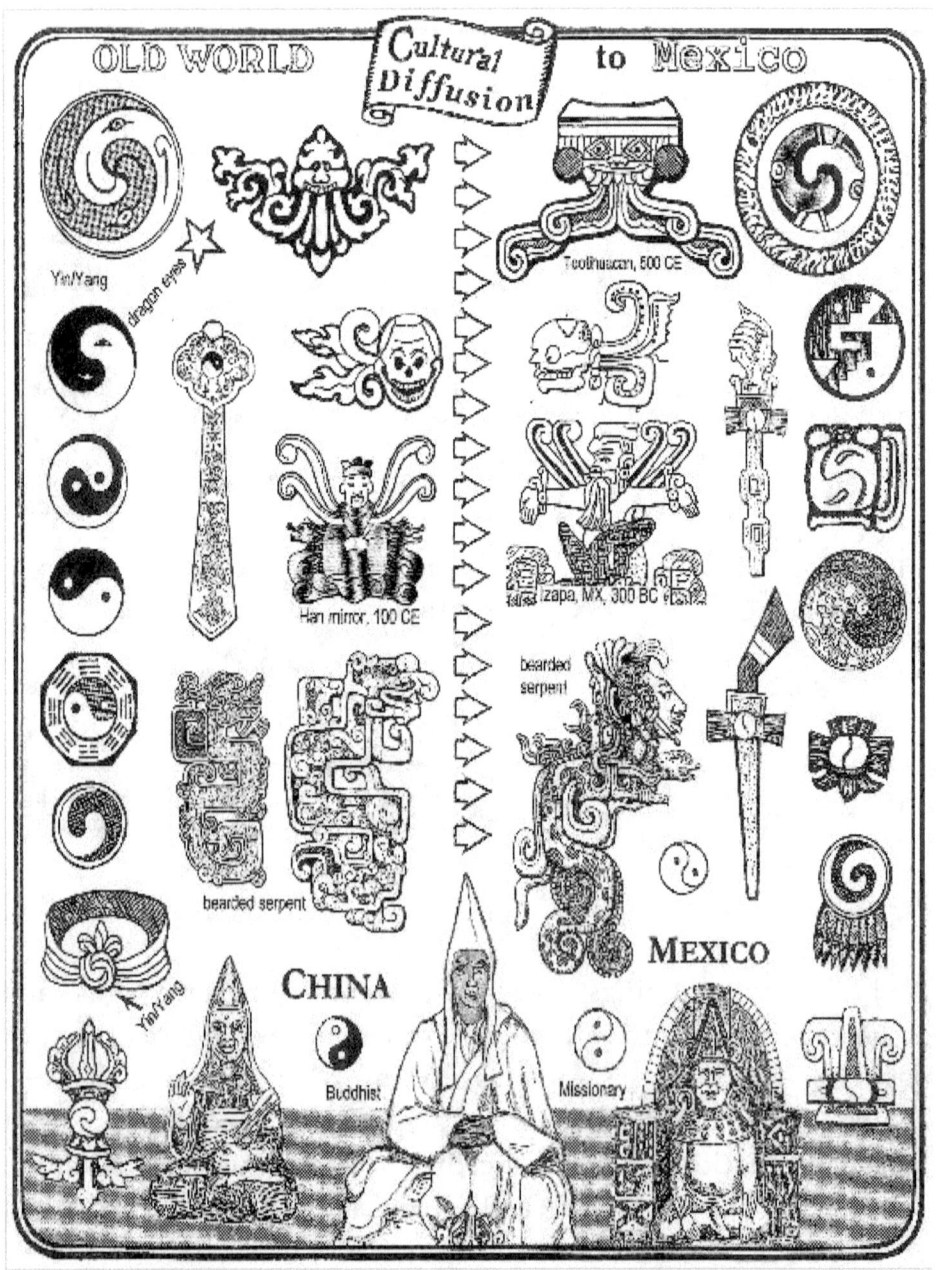

There is a bunch of scientific-speak in the above, but what it boils down to is that we now are beginning to understand that ancient man, even though we still wish to consider him to be 'ignorant or uneducated' was able to cross the oceans and trade goods back and forth well before accepted science tells us he could. Recently, realization has been growing among up-to-date scholars that voyagers using simple technology could have reached the New World millennia ago. Over 40 years ago, archaeologist G. Bushnell (in 1961) granted that there was nothing physically impossible about vessels coasting round the North Pacific at any time after 8000 BC. Since then, J. Fladmark has argued repeatedly for a similar thesis (in papers printed in 1979; 1983; 1986). Noted skeptic Ronald Dixon considered it "not unreasonable" (in a report printed in 1993) to assume that watercraft were capable of moving along the coast from Asia some 13,000 years ago. Six years later, in 1999 he had changed that estimate to 16,000 years ago.

Nowadays, the coastal voyaging position is supported more and more often. In 2000, a respected archaeologist, Dennis Stanford of the Smithsonian, even proposed that Late Paleolithic (Solutrean) hunting people from Western Europe had made their way around the ice-bound edge of the North Atlantic to settle in Late Pleistocene North America.

Support has continued more restrained for the idea of voyages directly across the Pacific. The hypothesis put forward 40 years ago, that voyagers bearing ceramics of the Jomon culture of Japan reached Ecuador around 3000 BC, was accepted by a number of prominent archaeologists but with some hedging. Edwards (1965; 1969) and Doran (1971; 1978) presented many details about the nautical capability of Chinese sea-going rafts and made patent that the rafts of coastal Peru and Ecuador were explicitly parallel in form and capability to those of China, Indochina, and India. The work of Edwards and Doran has been readily available but widely ignored.

There is no question that those rafts (more accurately 'ships') were capable of direct transpacific voyages. Although the date for historical documents on these Chinese and Southeast Asian ocean-going vessels only goes back to the 1st century BC, the craft could easily prove to be much.

In Peru, balsa rafts were in use along the shore by 2500 BC and ocean-going craft well before the 1st century BC (Norton 1987). Alsar (1973; 1974) demonstrated the feasibility of crossing the Pacific from east to west by sailing a fleet of three Ecuadorean-built rafts with a crew of 12 over 9,200 miles to Australia (the rafts even exchanged crew members at rendezvous points en route). Various forms of such rafts, in addition to large canoes, were used throughout much of Oceania (Clissold 1959). Our present state of knowledge about ancient nautics does not rule out voyages that could account for the early presence of corn and other crops, in Asia, Africa and the Americas.

Well, there you have it, corn helps to prove that there was indeed significant contact and trade between the Old World and the New World well before the much-touted voyage of Christopher Columbus.

Chapter 4: Corn In the Old World

In the last chapter I argued that corn was in the Old World prior to the voyage of Columbus. But that being said, it does not mean that the Europeans of the time were all aware of maize. For many it **was** a new discovery, it was a strange and exotic plant from a fare away land that most of them could not imagine. So, for most of western civilization, the story of corn actually did begin in 1492 when Columbus's men discovered this new grain in Cuba. An American native, it was exported to Europe rather than being imported, as were other major grains.

Like most early history, there is some uncertainty as to when corn first went to Europe. Some say it went back with Columbus to Spain, while others report that it was not returned to Spain until the second or third visit of Columbus to the Americas. The word "corn," as I have explained, has many different meanings depending on what country you are in. Corn in the United States is also called maize or Indian corn by the rest of the English-speaking world. In most countries, corn means the leading crop grown in a certain district. Corn in England means wheat; in Scotland and Ireland, it refers to oats. Corn mentioned in the Bible probably refers to wheat or more likely, barley.

At first, corn was only a garden curiosity in Europe, but it soon began to be recognized as a valuable food crop. Within a few years, it spread throughout France, Italy, and all of southeastern Europe and northern Africa. By 1575, it was making its way into western China, and had become important in the Philippines and the East Indies.

So, Columbus brought corn to Europe then? Sure, he did, but there was a small problem. Back in 1493, when Christopher Columbus returned to Europe with a handful of revelations and a pocket full of corn seeds. He had learned about many things during his travels to the New World, but few were as exciting as the promising grain he had encountered for the first time. It was unfamiliar; it was delicious; it was, as Columbus romanticized at the time,

> *"affixed by nature in a wondrous manner and in form and size like garden peas,"*

and it could, if they learned to farm it properly, help feed a lot of people in a very hungry Europe.

The only problem was that Columbus had left behind a fairly important bit of information. "He didn't take back the knowledge of how to process it," said Betty Fussell, the author of "*The Story of Corn*," which chronicles the grain's several-thousand-year history. "That might sound innocuous, but it probably changed the course of history."

Over the next few hundred years, most of Europe grew to misunderstand corn rather than embrace it. Meanwhile, across the Atlantic, the grain endured a different fate: It thrived, and eventually found its way to the very center of the American diet. But there was another chance for the Old World to embrace this wonderful American import. It was through the trade of the Phoenicians.

The Phoenicians have been trading along the coast of West Africa for over three thousand years. Their descendants are the Syrian and Lebanese traders who have settled in the coastal towns and cities. The earliest known European traders, Portuguese, arrived for the first time in Elmina, a town and the capital of the Komenda/Edina/Eguafo/Abirem District on the south coast of South

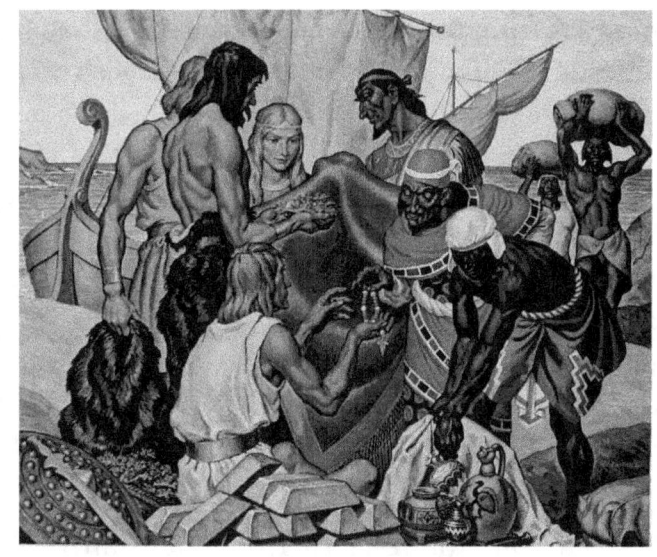

Ghana, In about 1472. They named it "The Mine" because it had so much gold for sale. Later they built the Elmina castle in 1482, a full **ten years before Columbus sailed.**

There was no demand for African slaves from across the Pacific then, because they did not know the Western hemisphere existed, and the sugar plantations were yet to be built. In return for gold, the Portuguese sold slaves from Sao Tome, located in the Gulf of Guinea to the people at Elmina. These slaves had to be fed.

Written records have not revealed what starchy food was being eaten along the coast, but oral traditions indicate that sorghum and 'corn off the cob' were grown on the Accra Plains, were fermented to make dokonu (kenkey) which is a Popular Ghanaian food, much like sour dough bread, made from fermented corn dough, and then used to feed the slaves. Later, maize was brought by the Europeans to West Africa from America where they had found it.

Maize was (and still is) so important in the Accra area, (Accra is a city found in Greater Accra, Ghana) that annual rituals are built around it among the coastal Ga-Adanbe peoples. Dokonu (kenkey) is a food that has deep roots in the culture of the Akan, so it is very likely that it goes back father into history than the European introduction of maize, although maize is the only starch ingredient in it today. In the famous Asante tales, known as Kwaku Anansi (Spider born on Wednesday), one of the popular characters is Dokonu Fa ("Half a Ball of Kenkey").

Spending a lot of time in remote villages for their research, most Europeans with their Western habits, take a roll or two of toilet tissue with them when they venture into the bush. Most however, when the tissue runs out, are introduced to the rural Akan method. After the kernels of maize were removed from the cobs to be made into kenkey or porridge, the cobs are kept to dry. Many of these intrepid researchers come back to report that the corn cobs make a much better product for 'tidying up' than does toilet tissue. So, it seems that there is much we can learn or re-learn from these ancient peoples, and I am not just talking about bathroom hygiene.

Below is a selection from an email corrispondence from one such archo-antropolgist, Dr. Lois Takainin, who I met online while researching this book.

"I asked my primary cultural informant and teacher, the Kontihene of Obo, if the name given to the Europeans, "Obruni," was derived from the Akan word for maize, which is "aburu." The two words sounding so similar I figured it must be the case, plus I thought the fine yellow hair inside the cob resembled the hair of Europeans. He replied, no, I had it completely backwards. The name Obruni was given to the European, and later when maize came, the maize was named after the European."

"When the European came, he brought new ideas and customs. Whereas the Akan would celebrate the day of birth as a personal Sabbath as did the tutelary spirits (Supreme God on Saturday, Mother Earth on Thursday, Ocean on Tuesday, Each river or cave on its selected week day), all these Europeans would rest on Sundays, go to their special little shrine house, and conduct their spiritual activities. Since in their books (the bibles) they

read special rules and regulations, especially to argue a point, the people thought that they were quoting new proverbs. The Akan people always quoted proverbs to make a point. The phrase "ne o bu be fufero ni" meaning "they who brought new proverbs" was given to the Europeans. Eventually "o bu be fufuro ni" was contracted to "Obruni," the current word for European."

"Later, when maize was introduced by the European, they called it aburu, implying that it was the food of the Obruni."

Dokonu (kenkey) is a delicious food made from maize. The wet corn meal is allowed to ferment for three to seven days, and then formed into balls and steamed. In Accra, Ga Kenkey is wrapped in the leaves covering the cobs, while Fante Kenkey made at Cape Coast is wrapped in plantain leaves. The flavour corresponds to those different wrappings during the steaming. The plantain leaves give a slightly bitter flavour, and since the wrapping is close to air tight, Fante kenkey is better designed for carrying long distances while travelling. The Accra kenkey tastes sweeter, reminiscent of sweet corn. White corn is preferred for making kenkey."

At the Reading University Home Economics and Agricultural research station in Weybridge, UK, kenkey was studied and it was shown that the fermentation process added protein to the kenkey, in a more digestible and available form than the protein of the original corn meal that was used to make the kenkey. Thus, allowing the body to more completely process the corn and so suck-up more nutrients from it rather than just having it pass through the system unabsorbed.

In another email, Dr. Lois Takainin related the following story that really puts us Westerners in our places!

"Shortly after Ghana's independence, in 1957, USAID imported large quantities of high protein yellow corn meal. The donors were dismayed to see that the corn meal was not eaten, but rather, was just fed to the domestic animals. When they were asked, the people replied that the reason was that the USAID corn meal was "Yellow Corn," and therefore fit only for animals. The USAID officials thought of themselves as culturally sensitive, so they went back to the USA and gave out contracts to research institutes and universities to develop a white corn that was high in protein. This took several years, and cost a great deal of money, but in 1971, their efforts brought a new white corn meal to Ghana.

*To their shock and surprise, the people just fed the new corn meal to animals. "Why?" asked the USAID officials. "Because this is yellow corn, not fit for humans," was the reply. The aid officials were miffed and mystified. To them the new corn meal looked white, and they knew it was nutritious. It finally took an anthropologist, specializing in West African languages, to solve the mystery. To the Akan people, in the Akan language, the word "yellow" was not a description of color as Europeans would understand it. It was an indication that the corn meal had **too much** protein in it. The protein would not ferment when making kenkey, but would rot, and not be edible. They needed high starch corn meal that would ferment to make kenkey. The fermentation process added twenty per cent more available protein to the kenkey than was in the original corn meal.*

We Europeans have much to learn about African culture, and especially we need to learn that we are not the sole bearers of knowledge, and should learn not to make ethnocentric assumptions. There is so much we can learn from these so-called primitive peoples! Good Lord we are arrogant."

So, we can see that corn was eaten in Africa, just that it is not eaten 'off the cob' as we Americans like it. This same thing holds true all across Europe too. Here in the United States, we tend to eat and enjoy our corn on the cob, in fact it is almost seen as unamerican not to eat it on the 4th of July as we celebrate our Independence Day. Hamburgers, hotdogs, potato salad, corn on the cob, watermelon, and fireworks that spells a happy 4th of July to most Americans. In Europe maize is simply not eaten as it is here in the US. In 2015 the people of the US ate some 203 million bushels of corn while the all the members of the EU combined only consumed 106 million bushels. That begs the question,

"Since Corn (maize) is the number one crop grown in all of the world, how is it used in Europe if not much is eaten?"

The cultivation of Maize in Europe is undertaken primarily to produce feed for cows, pigs and poultry (maize for silage including green-maize, grain maize, corn cob mix, maize coarse meal with husks). The word 'silage' here is one I had to look into and I learned that *'Silage'* is fermented, high-moisture stored fodder which can be fed to cattle, sheep and other such cud-chewing animals, or can be used as a biofuel feedstock for anaerobic digesters.

As well as being used for producing sugar, grain is also used by the food industry to produce maize-meal-products, snacks, cornflakes etc., and in pharmaceutical processes. As a renewable raw material, maize starch is used in the manufacture of paper and cardboard (it is an important additive in wastepaper processing). New packing and impact protection materials are produced in new extraction molding procedures from maize-semolina. Sugar-maize, normally marketed directly as whole ear maize, is finding wider markets.

In Germany, for example, the area cultivated with maize amounts to about 1.58 million hectares each year. Also, 78% of the maize-cultivated acreage is maize for silage, 16% is grain maize and 6% is corn cob mix. The acreage of maize for silage includes the relatively small arable lands used for maize coarse meal with husks and green-maize which is used only as fresh feed. It can be seen that there is a strong concentration of silage maize cultivation in the northwest and southern parts of Germany because many intensive fattening bull farms, partially interconnected with dairy farming, are located in these regions (North-West-Germany and South-East-Bavaria). This leads to a high amount of semi-liquid manure.

In France, as another example, many people would not even consider eating corn on the cob. If they eat corn, it's cold from the can and served in a salad with a vinaigrette. Serve a Frenchman whole corn on the cob, and he might well make a face and say,

"Ce n'est apte qu'à être nourri aux porcs!"

Which is to say, that it is 'only fit to be fed to pigs'. I even found the blog of an American chef in Paris who sent some ears of corn home with his French friends, along with the directions for how to cook it, only to have them come back a few days later to report that they could not eat it, it went straight to the sty!

The Spanish will use corn to make polenta, the Italians to make a special Christmas pasta, and the English to make muffins or a pudding, but the peoples of Europe have never learned how to enjoy corn right off the cob. So, there you have it, almost no corn grown in Europe is intended for human consumption, and even less is consumed as corn-on-the-cob. It is used in many processed foods just as it is in the US but the Europeans simply do not enjoy eating corn the same way Americans enjoy it. Too bad for them!

Chapter 5: Corn and Native American Culture

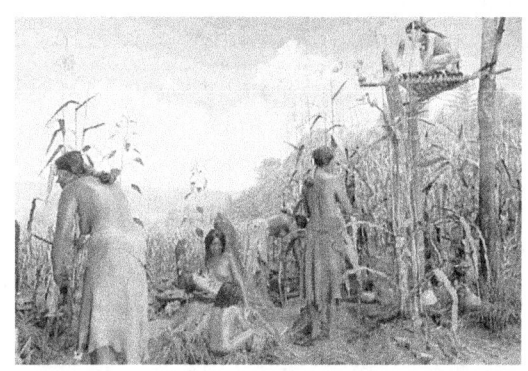

Native Americans were planting, growing, eating, and enjoying corn long before Columbus, Cortez, or any European settlers arrived in the New World and although corn is indigenous to the western hemisphere, its exact birthplace is far less certain. Archeological evidence of corn's early presence in the western hemisphere has been identified from recent findings of actual corn pollen grain which is considered to be 80,000 years old and was obtained from drill cores 200 feet below Mexico City. Another archeological study of the bat caves in New Mexico revealed corncobs that were 5,600 years old by radiocarbon determination. Most historians believe corn was domesticated in the Tehuacan Valley of Mexico. The original wild form out of the picture and long been extinct.

We now have evidence that suggests that cultivated corn arose through natural selective breeding of the Mexican grass we call *teosinte*. However, it should be stated that some interpret the evidence to show that cultivated corn arose through natural crossings of other grasses, perhaps first with gamagrass to yield the original *teosinte* **and then** possibly with some backcrossing of that *teosinte* to the primitive maize (which they believe to be extinct and as yet undiscovered) to produce modern varieties of corn. Whatever the case, corn as humans have been enjoying it for many generations never originated on its own. It 100% took the efforts of man to make corn what it is today. There are numerous theories as to the ancestors of modern corn and many scientific articles and books have been written on the subject. Corn is perhaps the most completely domesticated of all field crops. Its perpetuation for centuries has depended wholly on the care of man. It could not have existed as a wild plant, in its present form, anywhere on the planet. And it will not continue to exist with the unending efforts of man.

When the white people first came to America, they had never seen what we today call Indian corn, it did not grow in Europe. Nothing even remotely like it grew in England. The Indians raised it in little patches about their villages. Before planting their corn, they had to clear away the trees that covered the whole country. Their axes were made of stone, and were not sharp enough to cut down a tree. The larger trees they cut down by burning them off at the bottom. They killed the smaller trees by building little fires about them. When the bark all round a tree was burned, the tree died. As dead trees bear no leaves, the sun could shine through their branches on the ground where corn was to be planted.

Having no iron, they had to make their tools as they could. In some places, they made a hoe by tying the shoulder blade of a deer to a stick. In other places, they used half of the shell of a turtle for a hoe or spade to dig up the ground. This could be done where the ground was soft. In North Carolina, the Indians had a little thing like a pickax which was made out of a deer's horn tied to a stick. An Indian woman would sit down on the ground with one of these little pickaxes in her hand. She would dig up the earth for a little space until it was loose. Then she would make a little hole in the soft earth. In this she would plant four or five grains of corn, putting them about an inch apart. Then she covered these grains with soft earth.

In Virginia, where the ground was soft and sandy, the Indians made a kind of spade out of wood.

Sometimes they planted a patch a long way off from their homes, so that they would not be tempted to eat it while it was green. Those first Americans were very fond of green corn. They roasted the ears in the ashes (which is still an absolutely delicious way to enjoy corn on the cob today). Some of the tribes held a great feast when the first green corn was fit to eat, and some of them worshiped a spirit that they called the "Spirit of the Corn."

When the corn was dry, the Indians pounded it in order to make meal or hominy of it. Sometimes they parched the corn, and then pounded it into meal. They carried this parched meal with them when they went hunting and when they went to war. They could eat it with a little water, without stopping to cook it. They called it Nokick, but the white people called it No-cake.

When the Pilgrims came to Cape Cod, they sent out Miles Standish and some other men to look through the country and find a good place for them to settle. Standish tried to find some of the Indians in order to make friends with them, but the Indians ran away whenever they saw him coming. One day he found a heap of sand. He knew it had been lately piled up, because he could see the marks of hands on the sand where the Indians had patted it down. Standish and his men dug up this heap. They soon came to a little old basket full of Indian corn. When they had dug further, they found a very large new basket full of fine corn which had been lately gathered.

The white men, who had never seen it before, thought Indian corn very beautiful. Some of the ears were yellow, some were red. On other ears, blue and yellow grains were mixed. Standish and his men said it was a *"very goodly sight."* The Indian basket was round and narrow at the top. It held three or four bushels of corn, and it was as much as two men could do to lift it from the ground. The white men marveled at the workmanship on the basket and to see how handsomely it was decorated.

Near the pile of corn, they found an old kettle which the Indians had probably bought from some ship. They filled this kettle with corn, they also filled their baskets with it. They wanted the corn for seed. They made up their mind to pay the Indians whenever they could find them. The next summer they found out who were the owners of this buried corn, and paid them for all the corn they had taken. If they had not found this corn, they would not have had any to plant the next spring, and so they would have starved to death.

The people that were with Miles Standish settled at Plymouth. They were the first that came to live in New England. An Indian named Squanto came to live with the white people at Plymouth. Squanto was born at this very place. He had been carried away to England by a sea captain. Then he had been brought back by another captain to his own country. When he got back to Plymouth, he found that all the people of his village had died from a great sickness. He went to live with another tribe in the area. When the white people came to Plymouth, they settled on the ground where Squanto's people had lived. As he could speak some English, and as all his own tribe were dead, he now came to live with the white people.

The people at Plymouth did not know how to plant the corn they had found, but Squanto taught them. By watching the trees, the Indians knew when to put their corn into the ground. When the young leaf of the white oak tree was as large as a squirrel's ear, they knew that it was time to put their corn into the ground. Squanto taught the white people how to catch a kind of fish which were used to make their corn grow. They put one or two smaller fishes into each hill of corn, but they were obliged to watch the cornfield day and night for two weeks after planting. If they had not watched it, the wolves would have dug up the fishes, and the corn with them!

The white people learned also to cook their corn as the Indians did. They learned to eat hominy and samp, a coarsely ground and rather bland corn porridge, and these foods we still call by their Indian names. "Succotash" another native American creation givin to the settles is also an Indian word. Succotash is a cooked mix of corn and lima beans that is a personal favorite of mine. I even mix succotash with milk, cream, and clams to make a dish my family still calls "Indian Chowder."

The white people learned from the Indians to use the husks of Indian corn to make things. The Indians made ropes of corn husks, and in some places, they made shoes of plaited husks. The white people in early times made their door mats and horse collars and beds of corn husks. They also twisted and wove husks to make seats for their chairs.

Of all the plants that grew in America, Indian corn was the most important to the Indians. It was also of the most value to the first white people who came to this country.

The Native Americans living in the area where the English settlement of Jamestown was established in Virginia must have had mixed feelings about the arrival of these light skinned strangers in 1607. One of their first reactions was hostility based on previous experience they had suffered with the Spanish explorers that arrived along their coastlines. They attacked one of the ships before the

English actually landed. Yet the Native Americans soon began to offer food and traditional 'Indian hospitality' to the newcomers.

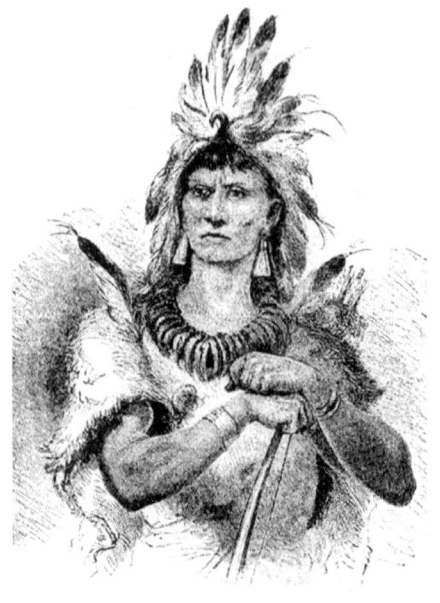

At first, Powhatan, leader of a confederation of tribes around the Chesapeake Bay, hoped to absorb the newcomers, as was their custom, through hospitality, offerings of food, and intermarriage. But this was of no interest to the early colonists, they sought only fabulous riches. The hard, cold truth of the matter is that the 'gold-mad' colonists searched for instant wealth so exclusively, that they all but forgot or rather they neglected planting crops of corn and doing other work necessary to make their colony self-sufficient. They therefore grew more and more dependent on the indigenous peoples for food. For a time, this worked out ok, but they soon out stayed their welcome.

As the colony's fortunes deteriorated during its first two years, Captain John Smith's leadership saved the colony time and time again. Part of this leadership involved exploring the area and establishing trade with local tribes. Unfortunately for those both the colonists and the Native Americans, Smith believed that the English should treat the locals much as the Spanish had: to compel them to *"drudgery, work, and slavery,"* so English colonists could live *"like Soldiers upon the fruit of their labour."* Thus, when his negotiations with the tribal leaders for food, or other necessities occasionally failed, Smith simply took what he wanted by force, at the point of a gun.

By 1609, Powhatan came to realize that the English intended to stay.

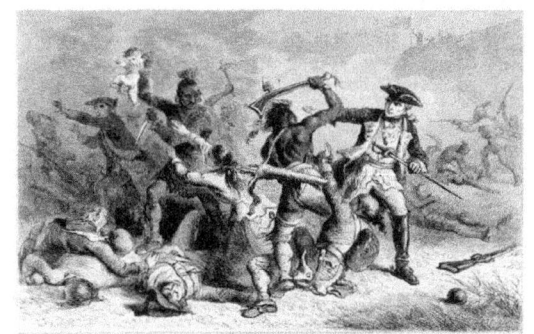

Moreover, he was disappointed that the English did not return his hospitality nor would they marry the tribe's women (an affront from the Native perspective). He knew that the English "invade my people, possess my country." Indians thus began attacking settlers, killing their livestock, and burning such crops as they planted. All the while, Powhatan claimed he simply could not control the young men who were committing these acts without his knowledge or permission. Keep in mind, however, that we know about Powhatan's reactions and statements only due to the reports of John Smith, who was hardly an unbiased observer.

In the next decade, the colonists conducted search and destroy raids on Native American settlements. They burned villages and corn crops (ironic that, since the English were often starving). Both sides committed atrocities against the other. Powhatan was finally forced into a truce of sorts. Colonists captured Powhatan's favorite daughter, Pocahontas, who soon married John Rolfe. Their marriage did help relations between the Indians and colonists.

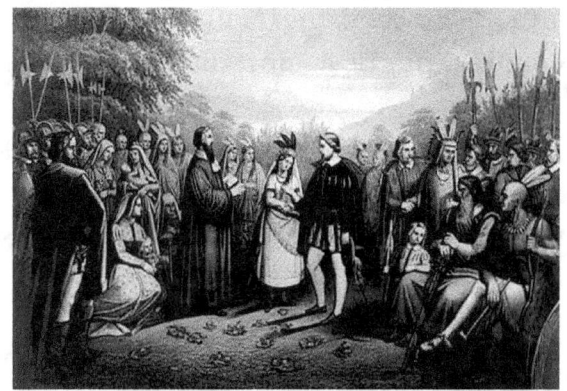

With the reorganization of the Jamestown colony under Sir Edwin Sandys, liberal land policies led to dispersion of English settlements along the James River. Increasing cultivation of tobacco required more land (since tobacco wore out the soil in just three or four short years) and thus, clearing forest areas to make land fit for planting was an ongoing activity. Expanding English settlements meant more encroachment on Native lands and somewhat greater contact with the tribes. It also left settlers more vulnerable to Native American attack. By this time, the Indians fully realized what continued English presence in Virginia meant; many more plantations, the continued felling of forests, the killing of more game; in sum, a greater threat to the Native culture and way of life. Many a war has been fought, on many a continent, for similar reasons. Even the self-proclaimed humanitarian efforts of people like George Thorpe; who sought to convert Indian children to Christianity through education, only made matters worse. Finally, the deaths of Powhatan and Pocahontas further hastened the outbreak of vicious hostilities.

The Indians, led by Powhatan's brother Opechancanough, bided their time. Pretending friendship while all the while they were waiting for an opportunity to strike the English and dislodge them from Virginia. In early 1622, they struck. In all, some 350 colonists were killed; Jamestown itself was saved only by the warning of an Indian Christian convert. One result was an ever-hardening English attitude toward the Native Americans. Another was a series of bloody reprisals against the local tribes.

Early on, corn was a peace maker but both the settlers and the Native Americans turned it into a weapon of war, burning fields of the plants to the ground in misguided efforts to keep it out of the hands of their enemies. All this led to was a bunch of blacked fields of useless dead stalks, rather than a life sustaining crop both could harvest and enjoy. It was a lean time for both sides.

You know, by the time the English arrived to form the settlement of Jamestown, and before any thought of war was in their minds, the natives of America could already trace the history of maize to the very beginning of time. Maize was the food of the gods that had created the Earth. It played a central role in many native myths and legends. And it came to be one of their most important foods.

Maize, in some form, made up roughly 65 percent of the native diet. Besides its divine connections, the natives had practical reasons for using so much maize. Maize was easy to grow. In fact, in this area, the plants grew and developed so quickly that two crops could be grown in one season. In addition, the plant was easy to harvest, was not too difficult to store in different forms, and had a variety of uses. The natives stored most of the maize they harvested. They dried it by placing the individual ears in the sun or hanging them in the air to dry. Nearly all of this dried maize was then "shelled," the kernels were removed from the cob. The natives ground these dried kernels into meal or soaked them to make hominy. The kernels of some kinds of maize could be popped over a fire.

The natives also ate ears of maize in the "green" from: raw and undried. The green ears were roasted over fires or the kernels were cut off and cooked with beans and squash. The natives had many uses for the rest of the maize plant, too. They used the husks that covered the ears to make baskets, mats, and moccasins. Green husks were used to wrap foods before they were placed in a fire for cooking. The silks, or "hairs," had uses such as padding. Even the stalks of the plants could be hollowed out and used as containers for such foods as maple sugar and salt or for medicines.

The natives referred to maize as one of the "Three Sisters," and they believed that the Three Sisters should never be separated. The other two "sisters" were squash or pumpkins or gourds and beans. Reasons that the natives believed the Three Sisters should not be separated undoubtedly originated in their myths and legends and stories that had been passed down through time. But practical reasons also existed for growing the sisters together. The stalk of the maize plant was strong and tall. It could provide support for growing bean vines in search of sunshine. Squash, gourd, and pumpkin vines grew thick around the base of the maize stalks and helped control the growth of weeds and the loss of moisture in the mound.

Thanks to the native population that they found in the Americas the English settlers lived, thrived and eventually gave birth to a new nation, "conceived in liberty and dedicated to the proposition that all men are created equal..."

COMPANION PLANTING THE OLD FASHIONED WAY WITH A 3 SISTERS GARDEN
corn, pole beans & squash

THE CORN SUPPORTS THE BEANS. THE BEANS ADD NITROGEN AND THE SQUASH SHADES OUT THE WEEDS

1) Plant the corn after danger of frost has passed.

2) Plant the pole beans when the corn is 5 inches high.

3) Plant squash seeds one week later.

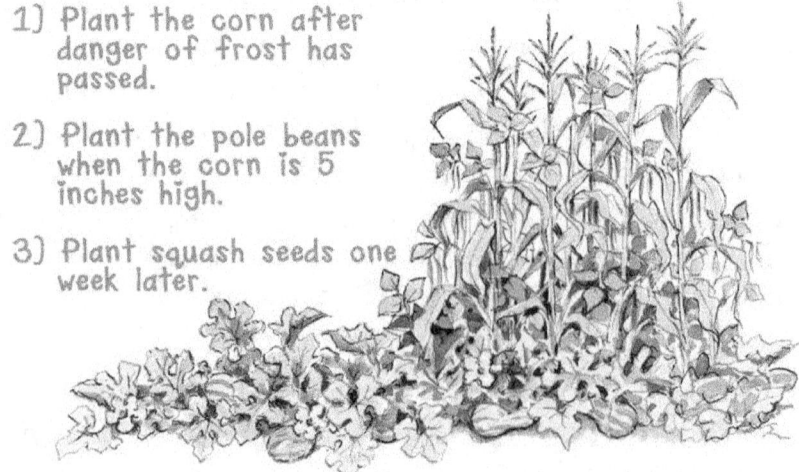

Chapter 6: Corn and Modern America

Let us make no mistake about it, people in the Americas consume more corn than any other people anywhere, over 16,000 million bushels every year. And in the US, we consume the bulk of that, almost 12,000 million bushels each year!

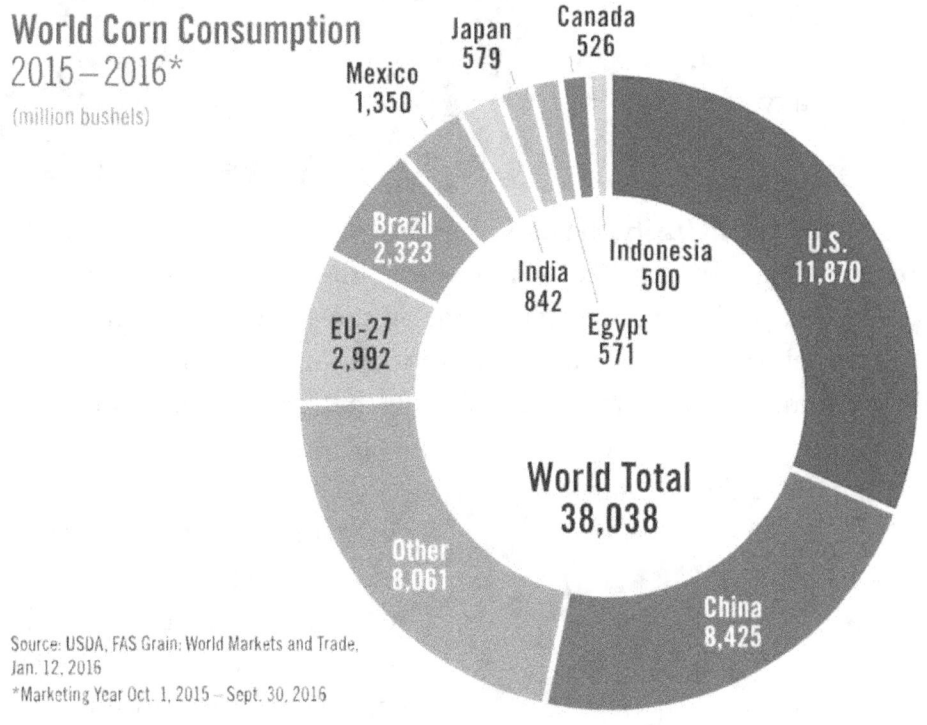

World Corn Consumption 2015–2016* (million bushels)

Mexico 1,350
Japan 579
Canada 526
Brazil 2,323
EU-27 2,992
India 842
Indonesia 500
Egypt 571
U.S. 11,870
Other 8,061
China 8,425
World Total 38,038

Source: USDA, FAS Grain: World Markets and Trade, Jan. 12, 2016
*Marketing Year Oct. 1, 2015 – Sept. 30, 2016

This being the case, we must look at the history of corn in America if we are really to learn anything about the history of corn at all. Corn is one of the most adaptable and varied members of the grass family. Sweet corn and popcorn are grown for human consumption but the majority of corn grown in the US is Dent Corn. But what is dent corn? What are some of the uses for dent corn?

Corn – the only important cereal grain indigenous to the Western hemisphere. There are three major types of corn cultivated in the United States: grain or field corn, sweet corn and popcorn. Grain corn is classified into four main types:

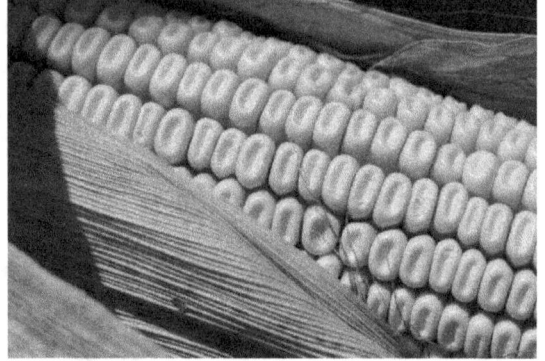

- Dent corn
- Flint corn
- Flour or soft corn
- Waxy corn

Dent corn, at maturity, has an obvious depression (or dent) at the crown of the kernels. The starches within the kernels are of two types: at the sides, a hard starch, and in the center, a soft starch. As the kernel ripens, the starch in the center shrinks causing the depression. Dent corn may have kernels that are long and narrow or wide and shallow. Dent corn is the most common type of grain corn grown in the United States.

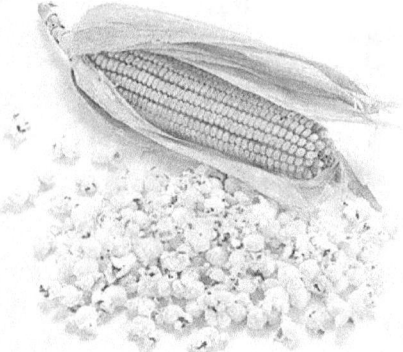

As mentioned above, popcorn and sweet corn are grown as food for us corn lovin' humans. But what are dent corns uses? Dent corn is used primarily as animal feed, although it is grown for human consumption as well;

it just isn't the type of corn that we eat right off the cob. Rather it is used in processed foods. It tends to be less sweet and starchier than the sweet corn varieties and is used in products that are either dry or wet milled.

Dent is a cross between flour and flint corn (more specifically, Gourdseed and early Northern Flint), and most heirloom corns from the Southeast and Midwest states are dent corns. Most varieties of dent corn are yellow, although there are white varieties as well which tend to command a premium price in the dry milling industry.

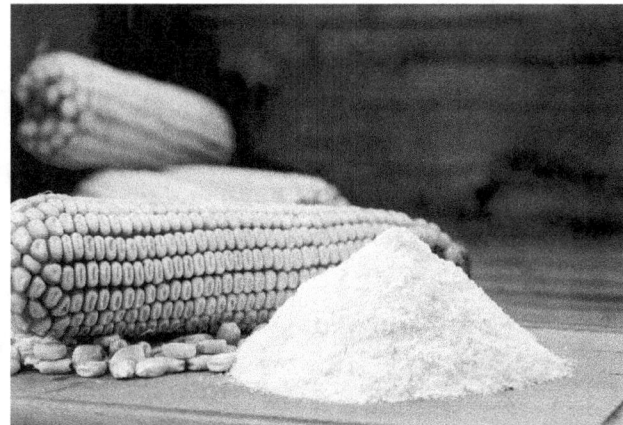 Flour corns are most common in the Southwest and are most often ground finely and used in baking, while flint corns are more common in the Northeast and used for making polenta and johnnycakes. Dent corns, being made up of both, are excellent for any of the above uses and are good roasted or made into grits.

When Old World settlers reached the New World, they found that the native peoples were dependent on this strange-looking grain. The European settlers had brought their own grains, which included wheat, rye, oats, and barley, with them. But they soon found their grains did not grow as well in the American climate as they had at home in Europe. Nor did they grow as well as the natives' maize plants, which the newcomers came to call "Indian corn."

The settlers learned to cultivate Indian corn from their native neighbors, who were growing large amounts of it. The newcomers even planted it using what they called the Three Sisters method of planting. Colonial farmers soon found that Indian corn could be grown with little skill or attention and quickly became very efficient at growing it. Some farmers could produce twenty bushels of Indian corn per acre of land. A hundred bushels of this life-supporting grain was enough to feed a family of six for a year.

Like the natives, colonial farmers also found that different parts of the plant had a number of useful by-products and purposes. They used its stalk and leaves for livestock feed. They used cobs to start fires and to fuel slow-burning fires. They used husks to make brooms and chair bottoms as well as to pad mattresses and collars for draft animals. Over the years, maize, Indian corn, or just plain "corn," whatever you may call it, has remained as important, versatile, and useful today as it was to the natives and the first Europeans.

Corn was the most important cultivated plant in ancient times in America. Early North American expeditions show that the corn-growing area extended from southern North Dakota and both sides of the lower St. Lawrence Valley southward to northern Argentina and Chile. It extended westward to the middle of Kansas and Nebraska, and an important lobe of the Mexican area extended northward to Arizona, New Mexico and southern Colorado. It was also an important crop in the high valleys of the Andes in South America.

The great variability of the corn plant led to the selection of numerous widely adapted varieties which hardly resembled one another. The plant may have ranged from no more than a couple of feet tall to over 20 feet. It was not like the uniform sized plant that most people know today. For the Aztecs, Mayas, Incas and various Pueblo dwellers of the southwestern United States, corn growing took precedence over all other activities.

The principal role of the corn plant during the 19th century was closely tied to the development of the Midwest. In the movement westward, corn found its major home in the woodland clearings and grasslands of Ohio, Indiana, Illinois, Iowa, and adjacent states. These were places where it had not been grown widely in prehistoric times. As early as 1880, the United States grew over 62 million acres of corn. By 1900, this figure had reached approximately 95 million acres; by 1910, it was over 100 million acres. The highest acreage ever recorded in the United States was 111 million acres in 1917.

From the beginning of records in the 1880s, through the mid 1930s, there was no significant increase in the national average corn yield. Yields during the 1920s and 1930s were no higher than those produced as a national average in the late 1800s.

It was not until the vast technological advances in the 1940s that corn yields started to show significant yield increases. Prior to this time, the highest U.S. average yield was recorded in 1906 at 31.7 bushels per acre. Following moderate yield increases in the 1940s and 1950s, yields shot up in the 1960s and early 1970s to a national average of 109.5 bushels per acre in 1979. In 2000, US farmers planted over 79 million acres of corn. More than 40% of the world's corn is produced in the United States. A bushel of shelled corn, by the way, weighs 56 pounds.

Total acreage is now less than in earlier years, but planting has increased in the more favorable areas of the Corn Belt. Iowa is normally the leading corn producing state, followed closely by

Illinois. As early as 1910, Iowa had 8.5 million acres of corn, which averaged nearly 40 bushels per acre. In 1935, Iowa had 9.7 million acres of corn, averaging 39 bushels per acre. In 1960, Iowa averaged 62 bushels per acre on nearly 12.5 million acres. In 2000, Iowa farmers averaged 145 bushels per acre on more than 12 million acres. The highest all-time record corn acreage in Iowa was 14.4 million acres in 1980.

Corn and soybeans form a major base of the Iowa economy. The combination of favorable soils, weather, and management know-how for the production of these two crops is rivaled by few other places in the world. Although few people are directly involved in the production of these major crops, many jobs are associated with this industry. Industries involved in crop processing, marketing, production of farm machinery and other farm inputs exist because of our ability to grow crops in Iowa. Massive livestock industries also depend on feed produced from Iowa soils. During the mid-1960s, about 75 percent of the corn was fed to livestock, 13 percent was exported, and the remainder went into human food and industrial products. By 2000, the relative amount of corn fed to livestock had decreased to 60 percent, 22 percent was exported, 6 percent was used for High-Fructose Corn Sweetener, 6 percent was processed for ethanol, and 6 percent went into other products.

Between 90 and 95 percent of the crop is harvested for grain; the remaining 5 to 10 percent is grown for silage. Of the corn fed to livestock in 1960, about 40 percent went to hogs, 20 percent to poultry, 30 percent to cattle on feed and milk cows, and 10 percent to other types of livestock. By 2000, these amounts had shifted to 29 percent to cattle on feed, 29 percent to poultry, 24 percent to hogs, 16 percent to dairy cattle, and 2 percent to other types of livestock.

One reference lists over 500 different uses for corn. Corn is a component of canned corn, baby food, hominy, mush, puddings, tamales, and many more human foods.

Some industrial uses of corn include filler for plastics, packing materials, insulating materials, adhesives, chemicals, explosives, paint, paste, abrasives, dyes, insecticides, pharmaceuticals, organic acids, solvents, rayon, antifreeze, soaps, and many more.

Corn also is used as the major study plant for many academic disciplines such as genetics, physiology, soil fertility and biochemistry. It is doubtful that any other plant has been studied as extensively as has the corn plant.

Today, the United States is the largest producer and consumer of corn — and by a long shot. Corn is in the sodas Americans drink and the potato chips they snack on; it's in hamburgers and french fries, sauces and salad dressings, baked goods, breakfast cereals, virtually all poultry, and even most fish. The grain is so ubiquitous that it would take longer to list the foods that contain traces of it than to pinpoint the ones that don't. "Our entire diet has been colonized by this one plant," Michael Pollan told National Public Radio in 2003.

But corn wasn't always so omnipresent. It took time for European settlers to warm to corn and, most importantly, a coalescence of fortunate events for it to sprout into an industrial behemoth. Until the 1800s, corn was eaten mostly by the poor. It was a cheap and prolific crop, consumed by farmers and fed to prisoners. And it was also used as a commodity. As Pollan wrote in his poignant 2006 book *The Omnivore's Dilemma*," corn "was both the currency traders used to pay for slaves in Africa and the food upon which slaves subsisted during their passage to America."

But then came the industrial revolution, and with it three essential technologies that helped propel the grain from the diets of the impoverished to dining tables all over the country.

The first was an iron plow, which allowed farmers to sow deep into the soil, and on much larger scales. The Midwest was planted with corn on a commercial basis precisely because of this new, simple but revolutionary tool. Two other advancements had an equally large effect, even though they touched corn production more tangentially. "One of the most important boons for corn might have been that the commercial farms in the Midwest grew up at the same time as the canneries and railroads," Fussell said.

Until then, corn was mainly distributed locally. But the rise of trains, which moved the harvest well beyond county limits, and the advent of canning, which meant it could keep for much longer, allowed farmers to grow with hundreds of thousands of mouths in mind. In the coming decades, the amount of land dedicated to corn grew incredibly quickly. It would be another half-century, however, until corn made its way to where it rests today; the center of the American diet.

Corn is what Fussell calls a genetic monster, because it's highly adaptable and easily manipulated. And there is, perhaps, no better example of its mutant-like qualities than what happened shortly after the turn of the 20th century.

In the 1920s and 1930s, scientists discovered a way to boost corn production to a level that was previously unthinkable. They bred hybrid strains that had larger ears and could be grown closer together, which allowed farmers to produce a lot more corn without

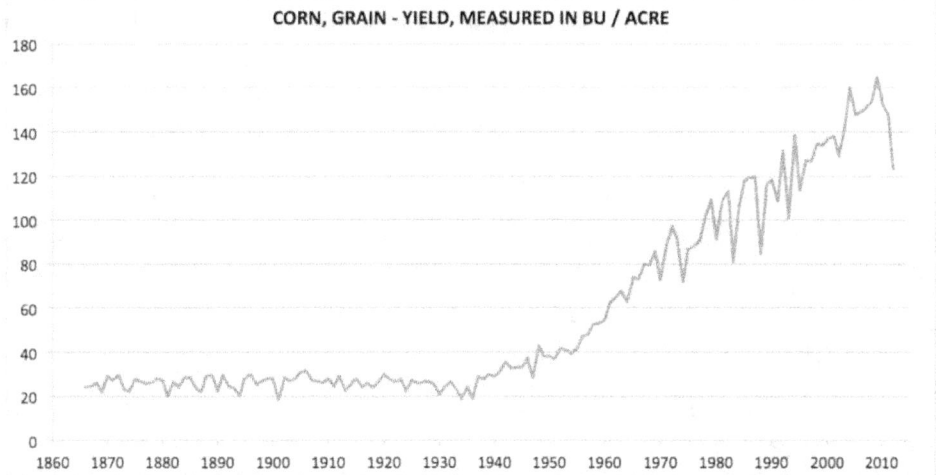

CORN, GRAIN - YIELD, MEASURED IN BU / ACRE

more land. The discovery, coupled with the introduction of new industrial fertilizers and more efficient farm tools, such as tractors, led to a thunderous rise in output.

In the following decades, "the number of bushels of corn per acre doubled, and then continued to rise each year," as Paul Roberts wrote in his 2009 book "*The End of Food*." Corn yields have risen ever since, with only brief interruptions due to sporadic droughts, interruptions that farmers are countering with further engineered corn. Advancements in farming technology and science paved the way for corn's ascent in the American food system, but what has allowed for corn to seep into just about every food Americans eat today is that, above all, it is inexpensive.

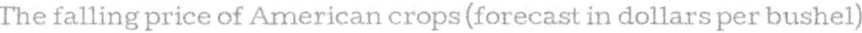

The falling price of American crops (forecast in dollars per bushel)

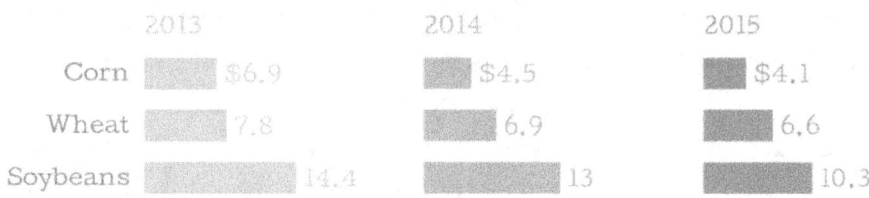

	2013	2014	2015
Corn	$6.9	$4.5	$4.1
Wheat	7.8	6.9	6.6
Soybeans	14.4	13	10.3

"Corn has and always will be cheap, because it grows everywhere in the world," said Fussell. At present, each bushel of corn costs about

$4.00, less than half the price of soybeans, and a good deal less than wheat. And the price is falling.

The most incredible thing about the corn grown in America today is how little of it we actually eat. As much as we Americans love our corn less than 10 percent of the corn used in the United States is directly ingested by humans. The bulk is either turned into ethanol, for use as fuel, or fed to the hundreds of millions of animals we raise. Cows, chickens, pigs and even fish, which are fed pellets made largely of corn, eat several times the amount of the grain consumed by people each year.

The relative cheapness of corn and general usefulness of it as a form of energy, both for living animals and living, more generally, have proved important enough that the government subsidizes its production to the tune of some $4.5 billion each year. The result is a perpetuation of ambitious growing goals:

> **Farmers, realizing that the more efficient they are, the more money they will get, grow more and more corn. The more corn there is, the lower its price, and the greater the incentive to use it in as many ways as possible.**

To talk about corn without talking about the different varieties would be to overlook an important facet of its ubiquity in the United States. There are many types, but the most commonly eaten forms can be divided into three general categories. The first, which is perhaps the most romanticized, is sweet corn. Sweet corn is what Americans grill in the summer, and boil or bake during the rest of the year. It's eaten on the cob. It gets stuck in your teeth. And it accounts for only about 1 percent of the corn grown in America. Flint corn, which has a soft center and harder outer shell, is what most people know as popcorn. It became popular in the 1960s after Jiffy

Pop, which cooked the kernels in aluminum foil on the stovetop, was introduced, and rose further in the 1970s and 1980s, shortly after the introduction of the microwave. Today, much like sweet corn, flint accounts for a steady but comparatively insignificant portion of the U.S. corn crop. And then there's dent corn, a.k.a. field corn, the most important kinds. It accounts for the vast majority of corn grown in America today, as well as the vast majority of the corn Americans eat. It's in most animals we eat, because it's fed to most animals we raise for slaughter; it's in most of the beverages we drink, because high-fructose corn syrup, which is derived from flint corn, is the most commonly used commercial sweetener; it's even in our cheese, because our cows munch on it instead of grazing on grass. It's largely invisible, in other words, but also virtually inseparable from the American diet.

"People have this kind of nostalgic understanding of corn," said Fussell. "They think of corn on the cob and popcorn. But the truth is that field corn is what we are really talking about when we talk about the dominance of corn in the United States."

"It's in almost every product in the supermarket today," she said. "That's no exaggeration." In many ways, Europe still scoffs at the grain that defines the American food system. The Old World is a wheat culture, Fussell says. But the truth is that corn's ubiquity in the United States has, in turn, boosted its popularity elsewhere. American-style processed food, which almost always relies on corn, touches countries all around the globe. This is why, globally speaking, yearly corn consumption is on the rise!

This may be a good place for me to ask what many consider a very strange question…

Did you know you eat <u>mutant atomic corn</u>?

It's true! In the atom bomb test conducted in the Bikini Atoll in 1946, a number of plant seeds were put in target ships that were located at various distances within the blast area so as to see what effect radiation might have on plant mutations. Common old field corn was one of these seeds exposed to the nuclear blast radiation, and guess what? It mutated!

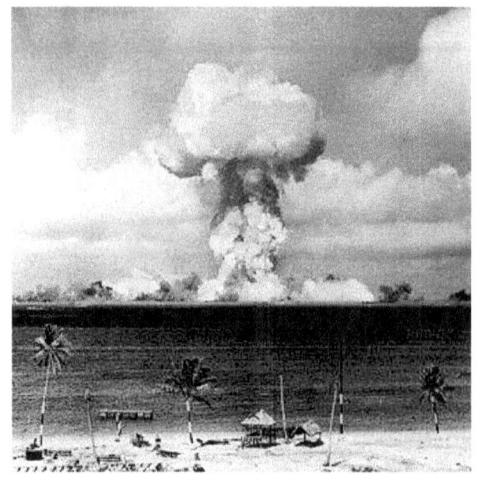

In the 1950's, at an experimental farm in Arcadia, California, Caltech biologists produced some of the world's weirdest corn crops. They grew dwarf corn just a few inches high, plants without silks or kernels, plants with intricately twisted leaves and no ears at all, plants that would wither in the noonday sun, and even plants that gave off a ghostly blue glow under a black light. These freak plants were in fact, descendants of those corn seeds which were exposed in the Bikini island atom bomb test.

Studying the plants was helpful in many fundamental studies of heredity and transmitted traits, but the Caltech biologists were really using them to study the effects of radiation on food crop seeds and indirectly on human beings. One day one of the researchers tasted some of the 'atomic' corn and found some kernels to be very sweet and delicious. He selected **these** seeds to plant and sampled the results. He would repeat this process, selecting the kernels that best fit the results he was after and before long he had bred a pale white

variety of super-sweet corn that was marketed to American consumers who ate it up! Literally, Americans consume 200% more corn (mainly the super sweet corn) today than our great grandparents ever did! To my mind the most incredible part about this is that if you have ever eaten modern sweet corn (and who hasn't) then you have eaten the results of atom bomb exposed corn seeds! *Ninety-five percent of all corn sold in US supermarkets contain the mutated genes form the atomic tests!*
So, yes, we have no doubt, all eaten 'Mutant Corn!'

Looking at U.S. Government Document AD473888, *"Effects of an Atomic Bomb Explosion on Corn Seeds,"* a report written in 1951 and classified as top secret at the time, (but which was declassified in 1997), one learns that the report covered the confidential work of genetic researchers who were growing and studying the "nuclear maize". It explains in detail how after growing and planting generation after generation of the corn they were able to raise the sugar level to where it is today.

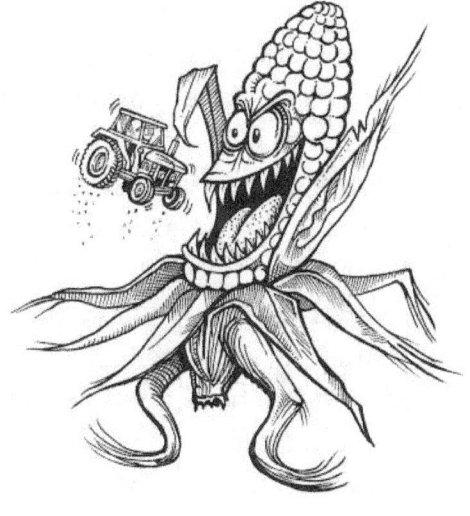

Before this atom bomb exposure experiment there was no such thing as the 'mutant-monstrous' super sweet corn we know today, but corn mutations in atomic bomb test samples produced corn with a significantly higher sugar content than the old field corn which ran around 5%-6% sugar. Some of the field corn varieties tested produced 12%-14% sugar after radiation exposure. With selective breeding by corn pathologists we now have sweet corn varieties with sugar contents of up to 44%! It has reached the point that you get more sugar in a large ear of white super-sweet corn than you do in a ***Baby Ruth candy bar (39% sugar) or a common glazed donut (41% sugar)!***

The tests exposing seeds to atom bomb blast radiation was code named **"OPERATION CROSSROADS."** Looking back on it, the choice of code name seems awfully ironic to me! The history of corn should serve as a cautionary tale reminding us that the unintended results of our actions are never foreseen, anticipated or easily corrected.

Many other books have been written on the history of corn so we know well what has happened over the centuries to this food source. Even knowing this, corn continues to be one of the most 'fiddled' with foods while remaining one of the most important crops in the world. And yes, we still continue to make the same mistakes!

An organization called the Corn Genetics Coop Stock Center is operated by the USDA and is located at the University of Illinois. Its purpose is to serve the maize research community by collecting, maintaining, and distributing seeds of maize genetic stocks. They also provide information about their stocks and the mutations they carry through the Maize Genetics and Genomic Database. Looking at the information available on their webpage one cannot help but notice that out of the thousands of mutant corn seeds sequestered in the Maize Genetics Cooperation Stock Center, the only varieties that have made it to our tables are the ones that are extra-sweet, soft, and either pale yellow or white in color, despite the fact that the center's collection includes kernels that are unusually high in protein, anthocyanins, or beta-carotene. All these more nutritious, phytonutrient dense varieties have been passed over in favor of sweeter, milder-flavored corn. The attitude seems to be "feed them sugar and watch them dance!"

A brief mention about Popcorn:

I absolutely love this stuff! First, the sound hits you; "pop, pop, pop," slow at first, then a firestorm of kernels as they magically transform into billows of crunchy white deliciousness. Next the smell wafts throughout the room, tantalizing your nose and your taste buds. By the time your teeth crunch down on that first bite, you're completely hooked. Popcorn is an irresistible treat. Try keeping a bowl to yourself during family movie night, or buying a small bucket at the movie theater. Before you know it, everyone is grabbing a handful. Popcorn is a simple, tasty treat on its own, but it also lends itself to a variety of toppings; butter, sugar, cinnamon, caramel, a sprinkle of smoked paprika, even chocolate! Popcorn provides a perfect canvas for your sweet and salty cravings.

So, what makes popcorn "pop"? The secret is in the kernel. Popcorn comes from a certain variety of maize that produces small kernels with a hard outer shell. These kernels cannot be chewed without a good chance of cracking a tooth. To get to the fluffy edible part, you must heat the kernel, which turns the moisture within into steam. When the outer shell has reached its pressure point it bursts, releasing the soft inner flake and creating what we recognize as popcorn. The popcorn variety of maize was domesticated by Pre-Columbian indigenous peoples by 5000 BC. It is a small and harder form of flint corn, most commonly found in white or yellow kernels. The stalks produce several ears at a time, though they are smaller and yield less corn than other maize varieties. The "pop" is not limited exclusively to this type of maize, but the flake of other types is smaller by comparison. Popcorn likely arrived in the American

Southwest over 2500 years ago, but was not found growing east of the Mississippi until the early 1800s due to botanical and environmental factors. Today the Midwest is famous for its "Corn Belt," but prior to the introduction of the steel plow during the 19th century, soil conditions there were not suitable for growing corn.

Evidence of popcorn's first "pop" did not appear until the 1820s, when it was sold throughout the eastern United States under the names Pearl or Nonpareil. Its popularity quickly began to spread throughout the South and by the 1840s popcorn had started to gain a foothold in America. Prestigious literary magazines like New York's *Knickerbocker* and the *Yale Literary Magazine* began referencing popcorn. By 1848, the word "popcorn" was included in John Russell Bartlett's *Dictionary of Americanisms*. Bartlett claimed that the name was derived from "the noise it makes on bursting open."

One of the earliest recipes for popping corn came from Daniel Browne during the 1840s. His method required one to "Take a grill, a half pint, or more of Valparaiso or Pop Corn, and put in a frying-pan, slightly buttered, or rubbed with lard. Hold the pan over a fire so as constantly to stir or shake the corn within, and in a few minutes each kernel will pop, or turn inside out." He adds that salt or sugar can be added while the popcorn is still hot. The problem with this method was that butter tended to burn before reaching a high enough temperature and lard produced popcorn that was soaked with grease. It wasn't until the second half of the nineteenth century that an efficient method for popping corn was developed. These newly invented "poppers" were made from boxes of tight wire gauze attached to a long handle; they were meant to be held over an open flame. Poppers offered several benefits, including the ability to contain the popped kernels while also keeping hands away from an exposed flame. Over the years, many improvements were made to the original popper prototype, which made the snack even more accessible to the masses.

As popcorn grew in popularity, it began to appear in all sorts of variations. Louis Ruckheim came up with the first version of Cracker Jack, made from popcorn, peanuts and molasses, during the late 1890s. There are several different stories surrounding how the snack first got its name, but it undoubtedly derived from a popular slang term during the era, meaning "excellent" or "first rate."

Popcorn's mass appeal was brought to new heights thanks to movie theaters. Surprisingly, theater owners were not on board with popcorn sales in the beginning. They thought it might create an unnecessary nuisance in addition to requiring expensive changes, like installing outside vents to rid the building of smoky popcorn odors. Hawkers, seeing the potential in popcorn sales, took matters into their own hands and began selling popcorn and Cracker Jack while walking up and down the theater aisles. The Depression eventually changed the minds of theater owners, and they began to view it as a small luxury that patrons could afford. Unlike most treats, popcorn sales actually rose during the Depression. Instead of installing indoor concession areas, theaters charged outside vendors a dollar a day to sell popcorn from outdoor stands. In 1938 Glen W. Dickson, the owner of several theaters throughout the Midwest, began installing popcorn machines in the lobbies of his theaters. The construction changes were costly, but he recovered his investment quickly and his profits skyrocketed. The trend spread quickly. Can you imagine walking into a movie theater today without the scent of popcorn welcoming you inside? I sure can't.

Recently the GMO debate has gained steam here in the U.S., particularly when it comes to corn. The majority of corn grown in the

United States is genetically modified. According to Jeffrey Smith, a GMO expert, the popcorn variety of corn has not yet been genetically modified. This means there is no genetically modified popcorn currently available on the market. Interesting that after all of these years, we're still enjoying popcorn grown from the same seeds our ancestors used.

And now a nod to the rather weird story of Corn Flakes...

Corn flakes cereal is a staple on breakfast tables all over the world. Today it is marketed as a healthy part of a balanced breakfast. But corn flakes were originally invented by a fanatically religious doctor as a way to stop people from masturbating. Yep, you read that correctly.

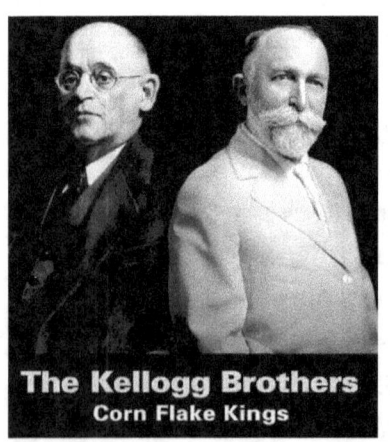

The Kellogg Brothers
Corn Flake Kings

In 1894, two brothers, Dr. John Harvey Kellogg and Will Keith "WK" Kellogg, were running a sanitarium and health spa in the town of Battle Creek, Michigan. John was the Superintendent, and WK was the bookkeeper. Among the treatments that were offered at the sanitarium/hospital for various ailments were hot and cold water baths, hydro-therapy with water enemas, electric-current therapy, light therapy using both sunlight and artificial lamps, and a regimen of exercise and massage. Among the more famous of the hospital's clients through the 1910's and 1920's were President Warren G Harding, actor Johnny Weissmuller, Henry Ford, Amelia Earhart, Sojourner Truth, and Mary Todd Lincoln.

Both of the Kellogg brothers were Seventh-Day Adventists, a fundamentalist church which emphased strict Biblical literalism and clean living, and their religious beliefs had a huge influence on many of their "treatments". The Adventists believed in maintaining the purity of the "body's temple", and forbade the use of caffeine, alcohol and nicotine. They were also strict vegetarians.

Dr. John Kellogg, however, took the Adventist faith in the purity of the body to an even further extreme. He was firmly convinced that sex itself was impure and harmful, and most especially the "solitary vice," the "self-pollution" of masturbation. Kellogg married, but never consummated the union, he and his wife had separate bedrooms, and they adopted all their children. Kellogg became famous across the country for his books condemning sex, promoting celibacy, and luridly describing the evil health effects of "onanism", which included everything from epilepsy to mood swings to dementia. "Neither plague, nor war, nor small-pox," he thundered in one of his anti-sex books, "have produced results so disastrous to humanity as the pernicious habit of onanism. Such a victim dies literally by his own hand."

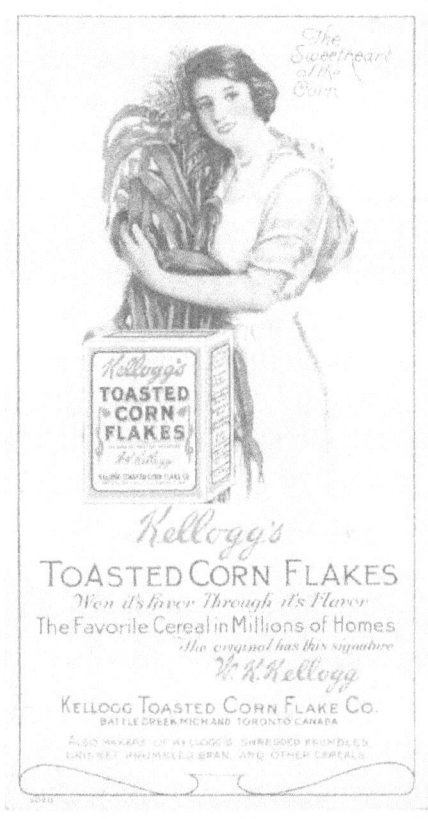

A part of his anti-sex and anti-masturbation "treatment" came from his traditional Adventist reliance on vegetarianism. Kellogg convinced himself that eating meats and spicy foods increased the desire for sex, and forbade any of them at his sanitarium. Instead, he prescribed a bland tasteless diet containing mostly whole grains and nuts. In this, he was following the earlier lead of Presbyterian religious fanatic Sylvester Graham, who had invented the whole-wheat graham cracker as part of a diet that would reduce people's sexual desire and stop them from both copulating and masturbating. Kellogg now attempted to make his own anti-sex food, by mixing corn meal and oatmeal into dough, adding nuts, and baking them into biscuits which were then crumbled into pieces. He called it "granula". Unfortunately for Kellogg, that name was already being used by another health food fanatic with a similar product, and he threatened to sue, so Kellogg changed the name of his concoction to "granola".

The Kellogg brothers also experimented with different types of bread, and with using whole-grain dough to make thin rolled sheets of toasted crackers. One day, after just having cooked some wheat for rolling, they were unexpectedly called away. When they got back, they ran the cooled wheat through the rollers, and each grain was flattened into an individual flake. It was, they thought, a wonderful health food. In 1898 they tried the same process using corn instead of wheat, and "corn flakes" were born.

John Kellogg immediately began serving corn flakes to his patients at the sanitarium, as a method of cleansing their bodies and reducing their sex drive. His bookkeeper brother WK, meanwhile, had less religious fervor and more business sense than John did, and thought they should add sugar to the mixture to eliminate the cardboard taste (a heretical thought to John) and sell it to the public as a breakfast cereal. After some arguing, the two patented their flake cereals and formed the Sanitas Food Company to sell them through mail-order, mostly to former patients of the sanitarium. After a time, the wheat flakes were dropped. But corn flake sales remained low, mostly because John Kellogg still refused to add sugar to the recipe to make it more palatable. Finally in 1906, in frustration, WK Kellogg purchased the rights to make "corn flakes" from his brother, changed the recipe, and set up the Battle Creek Toasted Corn Flake Company. After a long legal battle with his brother over the use of the name "Kellogg", this became the

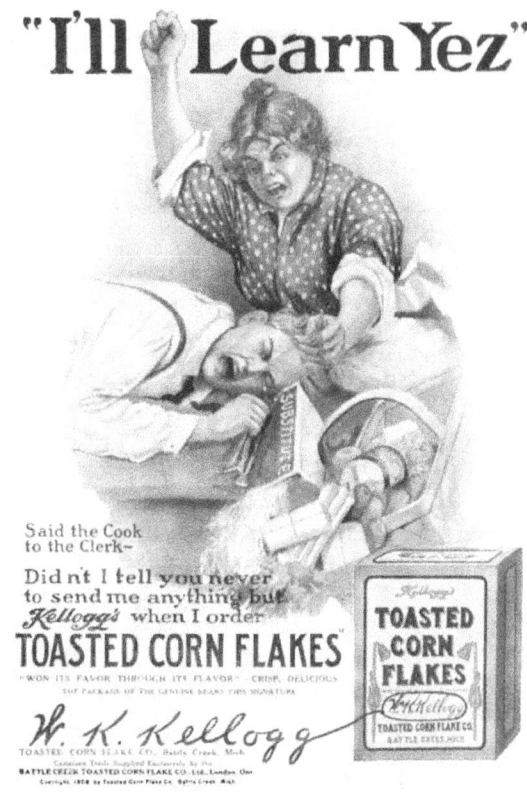

Kellogg Cereal Company, adding Bran Flakes to its product list in 1915 and Rice Krispies in 1927.

By 1930, the Kellogg Cereal Company was the largest breakfast cereal maker in the world. Its primary competition, the Post Cereal Company, had been founded by CW Post, a former patient at the Kellogg Sanitarium, who, WK Kellogg always claimed, had stolen the recipe for corn flakes from the hospital's safe. Today, Kellogg's Corn Flakes are the best-selling breakfast cereal in the US.

Chapter 7: Corn & GMO

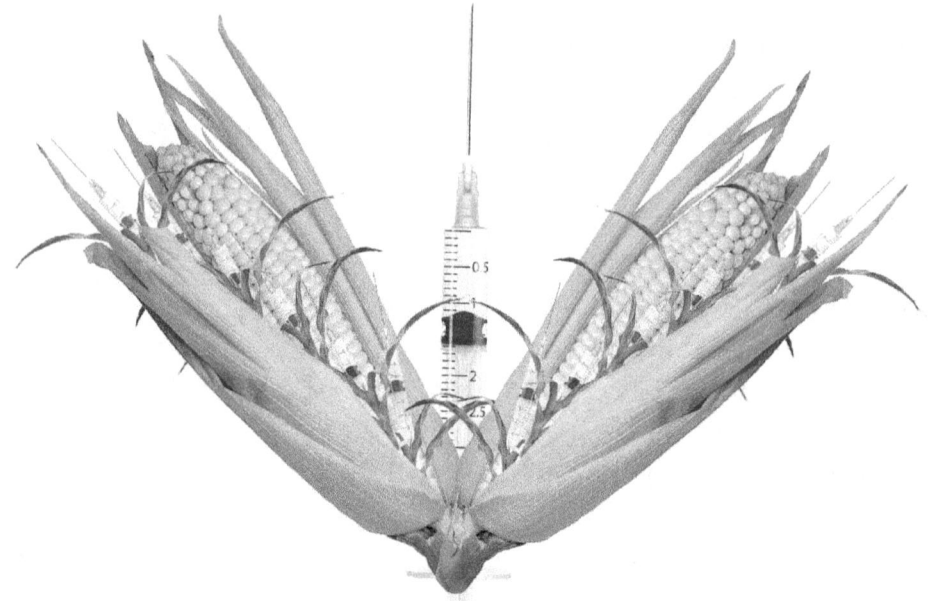

To begin this chapter I, want to make a few points perfectly clear...

First off, if I have to choose a side in the GMO debate I would stand in the anti-GMO camp. Not because I believe that there is some evil plan afoot to kill off most of the human population with "GMO Food bombs." No, mainly it is because of two points. First, I think that the ability to insert animal DNA into plants and plant DNA into animals is dangerous and just plain wrong. I do not want glow in the dark wheat thanks to phosphorescent fish DNA. And Second, the GMO industries constant battle against clearly labeling GMO foods. Let the American public decide if they want to buy a GMO product or not – do not hide it from us. There are actually a few more reasons that I will go into at the end of this chapter, but what I want you to know up front is that I believe that knowledge is power, we need clearly labelled products to acquire the information that leads to knowledge. GMO foods have been with us for nearly 50 years, and their prevalence in so many products on the shelves of every grocery store in the western world speaks to the point that GMO food is here to stay. So, I say, "Give us the information. I want to know, damn it!"

Look, ancient wild plants provided an astounding level of phytonutrients that are largely absent from our modern cultivated fruits and vegetables. For instance, wild dandelions found the world over contain seven times more phytonutrients than does spinach, and purple potatoes native to Peru contain 28 times more anthocyanins than commonly consumed russet potatoes.

In general, you can identify the healthiest super foods in our grocery stores simply by looks and taste; the more bitter and the more colorful a natural food is, the more antioxidants and other phytonutrients it is likely to contain.

But disease-fighting bitter or astringent foods, such as arugula, mustard greens, and Brussels sprouts are often avoided by consumers today; they were similarly avoided by our ancient ancestors as access to sweeter foods increased. So, too, was the case with colorful foods, which have slowly fallen out of favor in many cases. This represents a massive loss of nutrition!

The evolution of corn provides one of the most telling examples. The richly colored "Indian corn" now mostly used for fall decorating was once widely eaten and enjoyed. It contained far more disease-fighting antioxidants and less sugar than today's popular yellow or white super sweet corn.

Genetic modification is also making our modern food less nutritious than it used to be, according to a 2012 report given to the organization <u>Moms Across America</u>, by an employee of DeDell Seed Company (Canada's only non-GMO corn seed company).

This report offers a stunning picture of the nutritional differences between genetically modified and non-GMO corn. Clearly, the former is **NOT** equivalent to the latter. That is made even worse when one considers that *the very premise by which genetically modified crops were government approved in the first place was that they promised to be not only as good as non-GMO but exceedingly better!* That has turned out not to be even remotely true!

Below is a small sampling of the nutritional differences found in this 2012 nutritional analysis compiled by the DeDell Seed Company of Canada:

GMO vs. Traditional Corn

	GMO	vs.	Non-GMO
Calcium	14 ppm		6130 ppm (437 times more)
Magnesium	2 ppm		113 ppm (56 times more)
Manganese	2 ppm		14 ppm (7 times more)
Glyphosate (Roundup Herbicide)	13 ppm		0 ppm (WoW!)

GMO Corn was also found to contain up to 13 parts per million of glyphosate (the active ingredient in Roundup Ready herbicide) compared to 0 ppm in non-GMO corn, along with extremely high levels of formaldehyde, which is a well-known carcinogen. Perhaps it is no wonder that animals, both on farms and in research labs, avoid genetically modified foods when given a choice. They are not smarter than we are but they do seem to know better than we do on this account. Yet, in the U.S. upwards of 95% of all corn grown is now GMO Corn.

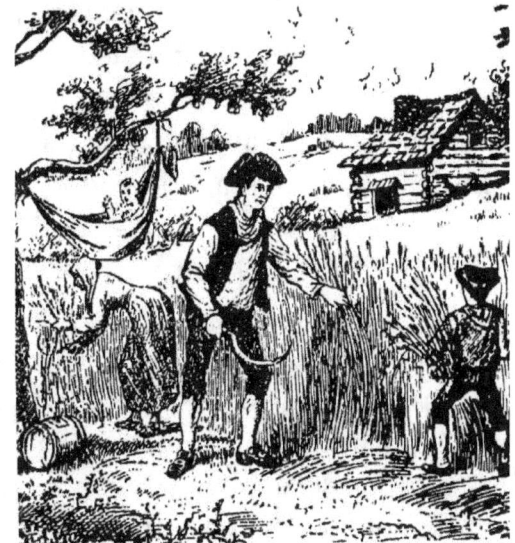

There is no question that when farming (or gardening), one wants to start with the highest quality seed one can get their hands on, this is just common sense. The trouble is that independent study after study is now showing that GMO seeds are _**vastly inferior**_ to most non-GMO seeds. However, I also believe epigenetic expression is every bit as valid in plants as it is in humans, which is to say that if we optimize the plant's nutrients through soil microbiology, we can improve the nutrient density of even GMO seeds. Better yet, if these optimization and enrichment techniques are used with seeds that have good genes to begin with you can far exceed even the optimal levels you could reach with GMO seeds.

OK, all of that above represents my true feelings and beliefs...
...on the matter of GMO Foods, but I do not want you to simply accept what I have said. So, I will now attempt to present a more unbiased view on the matter – presenting you with the information so that you can do your own additional research and come to your own conclusion.

The debate over genetically modified organisms (GMOs) can get brutal and often quite confusing, as unbiased research is few and far between. A lot of misleading information and impassioned arguments from both sides often clouds the conversation around GMOs, too.

A GMO is any type of organism, plant, or animal, whose genetic material has been manipulated through genetic engineering. While bacteria, plants, and animals can all be genetically engineered, you're probably mostly familiar with the GMO crops used in agriculture, like corn, soy, alfalfa, and cotton. The debate has largely centered around GMO crops because anything we put into our bodies that might impact our health can be a sensitive topic.

To date, scientists have engineered bacteria that produce medication-grade drugs, crops with built-in pesticides, and beagles that glow in the dark. While these are all relatively recent advances in scientific technology, humans have actually been altering the genetics of organisms for thousands and thousands of years, through selective breeding. Now with the aid of modern science, we can do the same much quicker by genetically modifying organisms, at the DNA level. Innovators, motivated by some of the world's most critical problems, have paved the way for GMOs — a path that leads to an unimaginable array of benefits, but also raises extremely important questions, concerns and fears.

The concept of "genetically modified organisms," or GMOs, has received a large amount of attention in recent years. Indeed, the relative number of Google searches for "GMO" has more than tripled since late 2012. However, humans have been genetically modifying organisms for over 10,000 years! Clearly, our ancestors had no scientific laboratories capable of directly manipulating DNA that long ago, so how did they do it, and how have GMOs become such a popular topic?

While our ancestors had no concept of genetics, they were still able to influence the DNA of other organisms by a process called "selective breeding" or "artificial selection." These terms, coined by Charles Darwin, describe the process of choosing the organisms with the most desired traits and mating them with the intention of combining and propagating these traits through their offspring. Repeated use of this practice over many generations can result in dramatic genetic changes to a species. While artificial selection is not what we typically consider GMO technology today, it is still the precursor to the modern processes and the earliest example of our species influencing genetics.

The dog is thought to be the first organism our ancestors artificially selected. Around 32,000 years ago, while our ancestors were still hunters and gatherers, wild wolves in East Asia joined groups of humans as scavengers. They were domesticated and then artificially selected to increase docility, leading to dogs that are closely related to what are currently known as Chinese native dogs. Over millennia, various traits such as size, hair length, color and body shape were artificially selected for, altering the genetics of these domesticated descendants of wolves so much that we now have breeds such as Chihuahuas and corgis that barely resemble wolves at all! Since this time, artificial selection has been applied to many different species and has helped us develop all sorts of animals from prize-winning racehorses to muscular beef cattle.

Artificial selection has also been utilized with a variety of plants. The earliest evidence of artificial selection of plants dates back to 7800 BC in archaeological sites found in southwest Asia, where scientists have found domestic varieties of wheat. However, one of the most dramatic and prevalent alterations in plant genetics has occurred through artificial selection of corn. As I have said before, Corn, or maize, began as a wild grass called teosinte that had tiny ears with very few kernels. Over the hundreds of years, teosinte was selectively bred to have larger and larger, sweeter and sweeter ears with more and more kernels, resulting in what we now know as corn. A similar process has given us large heads of broccoli, bananas with nearly unnoticeable seeds, and apples that are sweet and juicy. Although artificial selection is an ancient process that is still used today, most current conversations regarding GMOs refer to a much more modern process of altering the genetics of organisms.

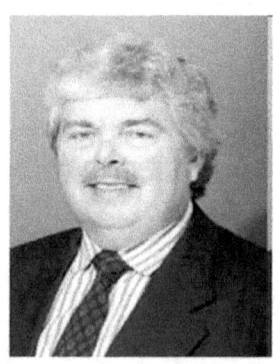 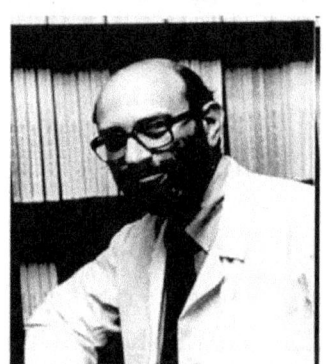

Herber Boyer and Stan Cohen Clone DNA into foreign cells; birth of recombinant DNA technology, 1973

An enormous breakthrough in GMO technology came in 1973, when Herbert Boyer and Stanley Cohen worked together to engineer the first successful genetically engineered (GE) organism. The two scientists developed a method to very specifically cut out a gene from one organism and paste it into another. Using this method, they transferred a gene that encodes antibiotic resistance from one strain of bacteria into another, bestowing antibiotic resistance upon the recipient. One year later, Rudolf Jaenisch and Beatrice Mintz utilized a similar procedure in animals, introducing foreign DNA into mouse embryos.

Although this new technology opened up countless avenues of research possibilities, immediately after its development, the media, government officials, and scientists began to worry about the potential ramifications on human health and Earth's ecosystems. By the middle of 1974, a moratorium on GE projects was universally observed, allowing time for experts to come together and consider the next steps during what has come to be known as the Asilomar Conference of 1975. At the conference, scientists, lawyers, and government officials debated the safety of GE experiments for three days. The attendees eventually concluded that the GE projects should be allowed to continue with certain guidelines in place.

For instance, the conference defined safety and containment regulations to mitigate the risks of each experiment. Additionally, they charged the principal investigator of each lab with ensuring adequate safety for their researchers, as well as with educating the scientific community about important developments. Finally, the established guidelines were expected to be fluid, influenced by further knowledge as the scientific community advanced.

Due to the unprecedented transparency and cooperation at the Asilomar Conference, government bodies around the world supported the move to continue with GE research, thus launching a new era of modern genetic modification.

There have been many controversies regarding GE technology, with the majority relating to GE food. While some critics object to the use of this technology based on religious or philosophical bases, most critics object on the basis of environmental or health concerns. For instance, a 1999 publication showed *Bt* toxin had negative effects on butterfly populations in laboratory tests, leading to strong objections of *Bt* use, but follow-up studies in actual farming fields confirmed the safety of this technology. In a different example, the economic stress of the poor yield of GE cotton crops in India over the late 1990s and early 2000s was associated by many organizations with a presumed increase in farmer suicides. However, it was later concluded that suicide rates were actually unchanged after introduction of GE cotton, and that there were economic benefits of GE cotton for most Indian farmers.

During the same time frame, public awareness of the existence of GE foods increased, and calls for regulation of GE food grew louder, resulting in labeling requirements for GE food in many countries. Today, 64 countries have mandatory labeling laws for GE food. However, the United States still does not have a mandatory, nationwide labeling law, although many advocacy groups are lobbying to enact one. These groups argue that labeling GE food is important for consumer choice and for monitoring unforeseen problems associated with the technology, (this is where I stand!). In contrast, groups opposing labels claim a law would unnecessarily eliminate consumer demand for current GE crops, causing steep increases in food price and resource utilization. Basically those opposed to labeling say that there is a PR hurdle that is too much for the GE companies to overcome.

Although the debate about GE food is active, and there is no shortage of opponents to the technology, the scientific community has largely come together and concluded consumption of GE food is no more dangerous than eating traditionally selected crops. This conclusion has not stopped businesses from capitalizing on the current fear of GE food. In 2013, Chipotle became the first restaurant chain to label menu items as "GMO," and in April of this year, the company announced the elimination of all ingredients made with GMOs, citing their "food with integrity journey." With cases such as this, it is safe to say the debate on GE food will continue for some time.

There are countless potential uses of GE technology in development. These include plants with superior disease and drought resistance, animals with enhanced growth properties, and strategies for more efficient pharmaceutical production. Likewise, GE technology itself is quickly advancing. Recently, researchers have developed a new technology called CRISPR, which takes advantage of bacterial systems to simplify genetic editing, allowing for easier development of GE organisms. (This tends to worry me a bit, and I admit I need more information about CRISPR – but the thought of editing DNA through bacteria is unsettling!) This technology could be used to expedite development of useful GE crops, facilitate disease elimination, or even alter entire ecosystems.

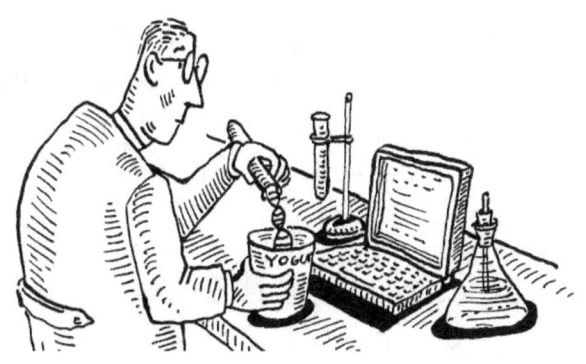

Interestingly, recent advances in plant breeding techniques may increase the utility and rebound the popularity of the more traditional GMO method of selective breeding. Indeed, new drought resistant strains of various crops have been recently developed using traditional breeding methods. In fact, these efforts proved extremely successful.

The United Nations predicts that by 2050, humans will need to produce 70% more food than we currently do in order to adequately feed the global population. Indeed, innovative approaches will be required to solve this problem, and genetically engineering our food is a potentially useful tool. As scientists look forward at ways to create better crop survival, yield, and nutrition, it is important that we remember where all of this work began, and give credit to the pioneers who have made these advancements possible. Our ancestors that selectively bred wolves to eventually develop Corgis could not foresee that today we would be able to genetically engineer corn to withstand pests, herbicides, and drought. What is the future of GMO technology that we ourselves can't foresee now? Personally, I would also ask, "Are we willing to take the risk?"

GMO foods are such an embedded part of our food system these days, but it's not difficult to think back to a time when food was simpler and, in my opinion, healthier. How did we get to the point that genetically modified organisms infiltrate so much of what we eat? In a recent issue of Rosebud Magazine, GMO expert GL Woolsey took a look at the history of GMOs. I present that for you here now.

1935 - DNA Discovered
Russian scientist Andrei Nikolaevitch Belozersky isolates pure DNA.
1973 - Recombinant DNA Created
The idea for man-made DNA, or rDNA, comes from a grad student at Stanford University Medical School. Professor Herbert Boyer and a few of his biologist colleagues run with it.

1975 - Asilomar Conference

A group of biologists get together with a few lawyers and doctors to create guidelines for the safe use of genetically engineered DNA.

1980 - First GMO Patent Issued

A 1980 court case between a genetics engineer at General Electric and the U.S. Patent Office is settled by a 5-to-4 Supreme Court ruling, allowing for the first patent on a living organism. The GMO in question is a bacterium with an appetite for crude oil, ready to gobble up spills.

1982 - FDA Approves First GMO

Humulin, insulin produced by genetically engineered E. coli bacteria, appears on the market.

1994 - GMO Hits Grocery Stores

The U.S. Food and Drug Administration approves the Flavr Savr tomato for sale on grocery store shelves. The delayed-ripening tomato has a longer shelf life than conventional tomatoes.

1996 - GMO-Resistant Weeds

Weeds resistant to glyphosate, the herbicide used with many GMO crops, are detected in Australia. Research shows that the super weeds are seven to 11 times more resistant to glyphosate than the standard susceptible population.

1997 - Mandatory Labels

The European Union rules in favor of mandatory labeling on all GMO food products, including animal feed.

1999 - GMO Food Crops Dominate

Over 100 million acres worldwide are planted with genetically engineered seeds. The marketplace begins embracing GMO technology at an alarming rate.

2003 - GMO-Resistant Pests

In 2003, a Bt-toxin-resistant caterpillar-cum-moth, Helicoverpa zea, is found feasting on GMO Bt cotton crops in the southern United

States. In less than a decade, the bugs have adapted to the genetically engineered toxin produced by the modified plants.

2011 - Bt Toxin in Humans

Research in eastern Quebec finds Bt toxins in the blood of pregnant women and shows evidence that the toxin is passed to fetuses.

2012 - Farmer Wins Court Battle

French farmer Paul Francois sues Monsanto for chemical poisoning he claims was caused by its pesticide Lasso, part of the Roundup Ready line of products. Francois wins and sets a new precedent for future cases.

2014 - GMO Patent Expires

Monsanto's patent on the Roundup Ready line of genetically engineered seeds will ends. In 2009, Monsanto introduced Roundup 2 with a new patent set to make the first-generation seed obsolete

Now, in my effort to present as unbiased point of view as I am able I want to take a look at the biggest concerns about GMO Food that really are not about GMOs at all.

Everyone from Chipotle to the neighbor next door that I almost never talk to, rails against genetically modified ingredients, and laws to label GMO foods are making progress in some states and many countries. But the laser focus on GMOs is often somewhat misguided, because many of the concerns people raise about GMOs *aren't really about GMOs at all.*

Do you find that surprising? I did, and researching this has been an eye opener of sorts for me. I learned that, "GMO" is the buzzword for genetically modified crops where the plant's DNA has been changed in the lab, typically by inserting a gene from another species. Technically there are other types of genetically modified organisms (living things), but no GMO animals are used in our food, though GMO Salmon are coming soon, and GMO bacteria are widespread but not very controversial.

There are serious problems with our food system and the way it is based on industrial, "mega-farm," agriculture. Subsidies support sugar-laden and processed foods while people on low incomes have trouble affording healthy, sustainably grown fresh fruits and vegetable produce. Meanwhile, needed farmland is being turned into housing developments, shopping centers and parking lots. Worse yet, massive amounts of pesticides and fertilizers are finding their way into the environment, and corporate giants like Monsanto have far too much power.

Passing around infographics about which GMO-containing foods to boycott, or putting tons of effort into passing GMO labeling laws, isn't going to do too much of anything to solve these problems. They will just make it easier for already-privileged people to buy food they feel good about — which may well be just as bad for their health and the environment as the food they're avoiding. Here's why.

GMOs Don't Always Mean More Pesticides
The concern: GMOs introduce too many pesticides into our food and in the environment.

The truth: Pesticides include herbicides (weed killers), insecticides (bug poisons), and any other chemicals (usually petrochemical or industrial waste based products) that farmers use to kill things that might hurt their plants. Some pesticides are okayed for use on certified Organic crops, and some aren't.

What does this have to do with GMOs? Two **different** things, actually, which GMO opponents sometimes get confused. One type of GMO plant *increases* pesticide use, and another popular type *decreases* use.

Herbicide tolerant plants can withstand sprayings of certain weed killers. Genetically modified "Roundup Ready" corn and soy plants were developed by industrial giant Monsanto, which (don't be surprised) is the maker of the herbicide RoundUp, chemically known as glyphosate. Farmers can buy the seeds and the herbicide, then spray their whole field knowing that the weeds will die and the specially engineered corn or soy plants won't. Glyphosate was popular well before GMOs, but now farmers have extra incentive to use it.

The bad news: thanks to these plants, farmers now spray *massive amounts of herbicide – far mare than ever before.*
The good news: (if it is good news) at least it's one of the less toxic herbicides. But this leads to a few bad things: weeds are becoming resistant to glyphosate, so farmers have to use more of it. In an attempt to solve the problem, companies are developing new GMO plants that are tolerant to other herbicides, so the cycle of **over-spraying and creating resistant weeds will likely continue.**

So, is this bad news? Mostly yes, but from an environmental rather than a health point of view. More glyphosate is being used, but it's not showing up on our food in unsafe amounts.

However, there's another kind of GMO plant: crops that produce their own insecticide. They're called *Bt* crops because they produce the same natural toxin as the bacterium called *Bacillus thuringiensis.* Like glyphosate, this was a popular pesticide long before GMOs came on the scene. You can buy both at your local garden center: the *Bt* comes in the form of bacterial spores that you spray onto plants, and is great for when caterpillars are eating leaves on plants like cabbage. The bacteria produce a toxin that kills insects who eat it, but even in large quantities the toxin is considered harmless to humans. Mother Earth News calls it "one of the safest natural pesticides you can use." It was lauded by the same sorts of people that grow their own organic cabbage—until scientists used genetic engineering to put the recipe for the toxin into plants. Now you'll find people claiming *Bt* toxin is dangerous to humans (it isn't) and confusing it with glyphosate (which it is not).

Not only is *Bt* toxin safe for humans, its use means that farmers are spraying less insecticide overall—a win for the environment and for farm workers' health, and a draw for consumer safety (since there weren't high levels of pesticides on food to begin with).

So, do GMOs increase pesticide use? Yes and no, depending on which GMO you're talking about. You really can't lump them all together and say they're good or bad as a group.

What you can do: We discuss pesticides on food on website at www.GardeningAustin.com frequently. To be honest, if you live in the US and you're worried about pesticides on your own personal food, the easiest tactic is either to grow your own fruit and vegetables or to just stop worrying and join those who believe that pesticides aren't on *any* conventionally-grown food **in dangerous quantities.** Meanwhile, buying organic means you'll still have pesticides on your food—just different ones. And, I don't have data on whether those are used in dangerous levels or not.

If you want farmers to reduce pesticide use in general, start supporting smaller, ideally local farms that are up-front about what kinds of pesticides they use, when, and why. Plenty of large companies and industrial farms have met the requirements to slap a "USDA Certified Organic" label on their products, so look for signs of a commitment to sustainability, rather than just looking for an organic label.

GMOs Are Unnatural, But So Are Plenty of Non-GMO Plants
The concern: We shouldn't be messing with plants' DNA. It's unnatural and could have unintended consequences.

The facts: We have been messing with plants' DNA for as long as humans have been growing plants. Archaeologists know that Native Americans bred the scrawny weed teosinte into the plump-kerneled corn plants we eat today. And 8,000 years before we figured out how to insert bacterial genes into plant DNA, the bacteria were inserting themselves into those very same genes; today's sweet potatoes bear their handiwork. And although many people see this as completely different from the CRISPR way of messing with DNA, many see no difference at all.

So, it seems, the question isn't whether we should mess with plant DNA, but rather how should we mess with it. Think of your DNA as an encyclopedia of cookbooks, and the recipes tell your cells how to make a person. Plants have a different set of recipes, which is why they end up as plants and not people. If you want a bigger or tastier plant, you'll need to find a way of changing some of those recipes.

Genetic engineering, as we mean it when we talk about GMOs, means that scientists are taking a recipe—a gene—from one cookbook, and pasting it into another.

In the case of *Bt* corn and soy, which I talked about above, they took the toxin gene from the bacterium *Bacillus thuringiensis* and inserted it into a soy or corn plant. In the case of the new Arctic Apple, the gene was cut from one type of apple and pasted into another. (Once the cut-and-paste has been done, you can breed or graft the plants in any conventional way. They don't have to bioengineer each individual seed.)

Genetic engineering is very precise in terms of the gene you're inserting, but there's no way to control where in the plant's DNA it will end up. If it gets inserted in the middle of another gene, it could mess up the plant's ability to make that recipe. That's why plenty of testing and screening is needed before the plant leaves the laboratory, to make sure it still functions as a plant and there were no ill effects. Sound dicey? Compare it to other ways we mess with plant DNA.

- **Mutation breeding** involves irradiating plants or their seeds, essentially vandalizing random recipes in an attempt to create a mutant super-plant. It's a technique straight out of 1950s comic books, and it actually works. (Most of the plants die, of course, but a lucky few get super powers like larger or tastier fruit.) It's how we got the Rio Red and Star Ruby grapefruits as well as todays super sweet white corn. If you're worried about mutant franken-plants with unknown changes to their DNA, *these* are the plants that should concern you. This technique is becoming more common as GMOs are falling out of favor in some countries. The extensive testing and regulation that apply to GMOs don't apply to these plants.
- **Hybrids** are more common, but still weird. When you cross two different plants together, the offspring sometimes show interesting traits that they may not consistently pass down to their own descendants. Some are even sterile, like seedless watermelons and other freaks of nature that people occasionally

assume are GMOs. They're not. Once again, you can find abundant examples at your local garden store: any packet of seeds produced by hybridization is required to say so on the label. If you want to grow a hybrid plant year after year, you need to keep buying hybrid seeds. The seed company makes them by hybridizing the two parents each season, like a dog breeder who keeps labs and poodles to satisfy the demand for labradoodles. *This* is why farmers were often buying new seed every year, even before GMOs.

- **Backcross breeding** is also used as an alternative to GMOs. This is where you find a gene that you'd like to introduce into your crop, but it's in another variety or sometimes another, closely related species. For example, in a project at Cornell, plant breeders crossed a butternut squash with a wild squash that was resistant to powdery mildew. The resulting hybrid was disease resistant but tasted terrible, so for years afterward they bred the descendants of that hybrid with butternut squash, keeping the ones that taste like a butternut but still have the disease resistance of the wild variety, and doing it all again next year. It's a time-consuming process, and is far more likely than GMOs to result in unintended genes ending up in the finished product, since you start with an infusion of thousands of genes instead of just inserting one. In short, if you're worried about unnatural DNA manipulation or the possibility of introducing unintended mutations, GMOs are just one of many methods that could, maybe, possibly, introduce a mystery mutation. (To be clear, we don't know of any serious problems that have come up from any of these methods; it's more hypothetical.)

What you can do: It's just about impossible to avoid plants that have been genetically altered somehow. If you're very dedicated, you could decide which methods you approve of, find the names of those plant varieties, and look for those when you shop for groceries or for garden plants. For most people, though, this should be a non-issue: just a glimpse of the bizarre reality behind how your food is (and was historically) made.

The concern: Monsanto, maker of GMO crops, is totally evil.

The facts: Agreed, to a point: Monsanto and companies like it are, in my opinion, bad for agriculture. To be clear, this isn't *just* Monsanto: we have to remember that Dow and Bayer, among others, use the same one-two punch to sell GMO seeds alongside their brand of pesticide. The big companies use market leverage and patent law to bully farmers into doing things their way. But here's the thing: big companies are controlling agriculture *for reasons unrelated to GMOs*, so a fight against GMOs won't really reduce the control they have over agriculture.

I really don't like that these companies own so much of American agriculture. But genetically modified crops only date back to the 1970s, and we had many of these industrial agriculture giants long before that. Banning or embracing GMOs is not much more than rearranging deck chairs.

The health, environmental, and economic problems of industrial agriculture have deep roots and can't be solved with a labeling law or two. Large-scale farms that grow corn or soy in **monoculture**, with an emphasis on killing native plants (aka "weeds"), are decreasing biodiversity (like the milkweed that monarch butterflies require to reproduce). Nutrient cycles in the environment have been disrupted: Instead of animal manure providing fertilizer for plants on the same farm, we have feedlots where "lagoons" of animal waste create health and environmental hazards, while hundreds of miles away, farmers cover their fields in synthetic fertilizer that runs off into nearby waterways, disrupting ecosystems and killing fish. In my mind this is a real definition of insanity!

Who wins in this scenario? Pesticide manufacturers, for sure (with or without GMOs). Many Seed breeders (with or without GMOs). Fertilizer manufacturers. Since the US government subsidizes corn and soy, farmers can sell these crops for less than they spent to grow them, which means consumers get cheap food (so long as it's made from corn and soy, which most processed food is). The companies that make the processed food win out. The whole system is kind of a wash for farmers (they would do fine with or without GMOs, and many are barely making ends meet anyway). Consumers like you and me? We get cheap food (yay!) but it's the least healthy kind of food (boo.) Not so much because GMOs are unhealthy but because the stuff you can make out of corn syrup and corn starch and soybean oil and soy protein **is *junk food and is unhealthy!***

Nathanael Johnson, in wrapping up six months of reporting on genetically modified food, lays out the real future that would await us if we could somehow ban GMOs:

In the GMO-free future, farming still looks pretty much the same. Without insect-resistant crops, farmers spray more broad-spectrum insecticides, which do some collateral damage to surrounding food webs. Without herbicide-resistant crops, farmers spray less glyphosate, which slows the spread of glyphosate-resistant weeds and perhaps leads to healthier soil biota. Farmers also till their fields more often, which kills soil biota, and releases a lot more greenhouse gases. The banning of GMOs hasn't led to a transformation of agriculture because GM seed was never a linchpin supporting the conventional food system: Farmers could always do fine without it. Eaters no longer worry about the potential threat of GMO health hazards, but they are subject to new risks: GMOs were neither the first, nor have they been the last, agricultural innovation, and each of these technologies comes with its own potential hazards. Plant scientists will have increased their use of mutagenesis and epigenetic manipulation, perhaps. We no longer have biotech patents, but we still have traditional seed-breeding patents. Life goes on.

In this view, in other words, **GMOs were a red herring all along.**

In fact, there are plenty of examples where GMO plants are being used for reasons other than profit, like vitamin-A-containing rice and protein-rich potatoes meant to alleviate malnutrition in vulnerable parts of the world. If we're fighting over-industrialization of agriculture, GMOs are the wrong battleground.

What you can do: This isn't an easy one. In terms of policy, here's a crazy idea: what if we paid farmers for taking care of the environment (protecting watersheds, maintaining preserves of native plants) instead of subsidizing every bushel of corn they produce? What if we expanded ways for people on low incomes to buy healthier and locally produced food, like the Double Dollars programs where SNAP benefits buy twice as much at the farmer's market than at the grocery store?

Back on the home front, decisions become clearer but (without systemic support) sometimes more expensive or difficult. Shopping from those local farms, like I mentioned above, is a tactic that works here too. You may have to change your repertoire of favorite recipes and learn to love meals that take advantage of what's locally and seasonally available. (But don't worry—there's more available than you think, even in temperate climates.) Consider a community supported agriculture (CSA) subscription for a steady supply of local food that supports your friendly neighborhood farmer. (Since you pay up front, you're reducing their financial risk at the beginning of the season.) Sometimes you can work a few shifts on the farm in exchange for free or discounted produce.

If you have space for a garden, or even a few containers, growing your own is a great way to make a dent in your food footprint. (Don't forget to look around you for community gardens, too.) There's a learning curve, but gardening can open your eyes to how food is really produced, and the real problems farmers struggle with: you'll find yourself dealing with weeds, insect pests, and challenges to fertilizing.

I grow a garden myself, and here's my full disclosure: It's about 99% organic.

I typically live with lower yields instead of spraying weed killers or insecticides, and I fertilize with compost or with "natural" items like blood and bone meal (much of which, I realize, probably comes from factory-farmed animals.) I do take the time to look for organic seeds, and I prefer both hybrid and heirloom varieties that pack the most phytonutrients in each final product. (For more information on Phytonutrients and their importance to our health, you can check out my website at www.GardeningAustin.com where you can find my *"Yes, Food IS Medicine"* series that goes into great depth on the subject of understanding, eating, and growing phytonutrient-rich, antioxidant-dense, fruits and vegetables.

I am not in favor of GMOs but I am a realist and I understand that they have been around for a long time now and I do not see them going away (some may call me a defeatist on that – so be it). Since I am convinced that they are here to stay I want clear labeling policy to be enacted into law. I want the information available so that I have the knowledge and am thereby empowered to take control over what I choose to put into my body and what I choose to feed to my family. That really shouldn't be too much to ask.

Chapter 8: Yes, Food IS Medicine

"Let food be thy medicine and medicine be thy food." This quote is attributed to Hippocrates. Another of my favorite quotes is *"Who said anything about medicine? Let's eat!"* which is attributed to one of Hippocrates forgotten (and hilarious) students.

Who hasn't seen or heard Hippocrates' famous quote above? If you have Facebook friends who are the least bit into "natural" medicine or living, you've almost certainly come across it in your feed, and if you're a reader of my Phytonutrient Blog, you will absolutely have heard the quote. Now Hippocrates lived a very long time ago, that is definitely true but just because an idea is old, doesn't mean it's good, any more than just because Hippocrates said it means it must be true. But in this case, it does and it is!

Remember, Hippocrates was an important figure in the history of medicine because he was among the earliest to assert that diseases were caused by natural processes rather than the gods and because of his emphasis on the careful observation and documentation of patient history and physical findings, which led to the discovery of physical signs associated with diseases of specific organs. He is also known to have been a great healer because of his knowledge of the culinary and medicinal uses of herbs and spices. But you know what? Hippocrates was not the only advocate for letting food be thy medicine. Throughout the ages there have been many others. Ever since man first climbed down from the trees (or, depending upon your view, plucked that apple off that tree), eating has never been far from his mind (survival has a way of prioritizing everything). The simple fact that sustenance equals life, means that food and health have culturally ridden shotgun throughout the ages.

"Good men eat and drink so they can live," noted Socrates.
"Eat, drink, and be merry!" commanded Solomon.

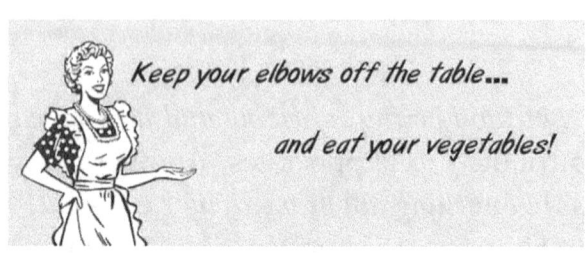

"You're famished. I'll fix you a plate!!" pleaded my mother.

In the days before medicine, food and drink was medicine...or at least it was seen as such. A browned apple for an upset stomach, chicken soup for congestion, champagne for septicemia (Pulitzer Prize-winning novelist Eudora Welty said her Mississippi father swore his use of the bubbly saved her ill mother's life). It was sometimes hard to establish cause and effect (Garlic as an anti-vampiric? Hard to find test subjects for that one,) and yet generations of pantries held foods sworn to bind, purge, ameliorate, instigate, invigorate...in short, improve one's well-being. And then came modern allopathic-oriented science, which until recently tossed nutrition—and its potential effect on both maintaining health and calming illness—into the compost heap. The reasons were myriad. Politically, no one had ever been elected on an anti-cheeseburger platform, so administrative pressure to funnel government dollars toward nutritional research traditionally was nil. Similarly, big pharma was scarce with cash, because they can't patent a food's natural properties. And from a practical viewpoint, studying food with its thousands of chemicals and nutrients is incredibly complex. By comparison, targeting and studying a single drug for efficacy in a double-blind model was far more straightforward and lucrative to both researchers and industry.

It took the American Medical Association until 2002 to reverse a long-standing position and suggest that adults take a multivitamin every day. Then again, many of its long-standing members had never been exposed to a nutrition elective while in medical school…creating a drug-oriented bias that historically expressed itself in both the clinic and the lab.

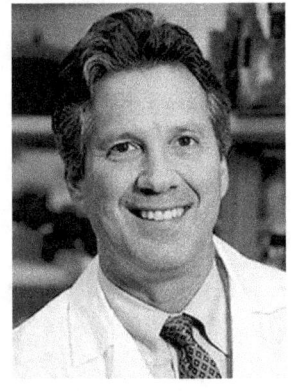

"I think for a long time the major directions in molecular biology—the ability to make genetically altered mice that could measure the impacts of certain molecules on the body—was totally not applied to nutrition," - Hopkins' William Nelson, director of the Sidney Kimmel Cancer Center.

That Nelson can speak of such research deficiencies in the past tense is indicative of a huge shift toward nutritional research in just the past 10 to 15 years. Again, I remind you that the information I present in this series, while in truth very old is now being backed by 21st Century science and research!

What then is the catalyst for this paradigm shift in thinking? Well since you asked I'll tell you what I think. We can't seem to shut our mouths, and the stats from the Centers for Disease Control back that up! With the exception of Colorado dwellers, more than 20% of the U.S. population is now considered obese. Given obesity's epidemiologically supported impact on cardiac, vascular, cancer, and diabetic-related illness, researchers are now branching out to uncover the myriad ways food and its micro components enhance or disrupt life. The sheer numbers of nutritional studies bear out this interest. According to Pub Med, such published investigations more than doubled between the 1980s and 1990s, and leapt another 71%

this decade. Part of the quantum leap in the last five years especially, is the discovery that chronic inflammation is slowly being linked to diseases including cancer, and that foods—from cloves to walnuts— appear to contain anti-inflammatory properties.

This critical mass of information even has a name. Called the 'Food as Medicine movement', it's a growing recognition on the part of many academic clinicians that to ignore the role of food and nutrition in health is to lose a valuable tool that can support (or perhaps even lessen or replace) many pharmaceuticals currently in use.

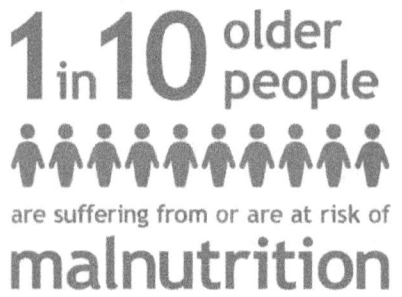

1 in 10 older people

are suffering from or are at risk of

malnutrition

"The perfect example is ginger," says Hopkins gastroenterologist Gerard Mullin, arguably the nation's top expert on the relationship between food and gut disorders. *"People who have nausea, or gastric dysmotilities or other GI problems, for them ginger is at the top of my list. It works the same way (the big pharma produced) Zofran does, which is one of our most powerful anti-nausea drugs. It works on the same receptor in the brain. But a lot of docs aren't aware of it."*

Similarly, food plays a huge role in how well people battle cancer. Researchers estimate that some 80% of cancer patients are malnourished, at the very time when chemotherapy often increases the body's need for proteins and other nutrients. Such malnourishment, if not addressed, can lead to a reduction of chemotherapy doses and ultimately poorer outcomes. Oncologist Bill Nelson says that the link between calories taken in—the so-called "caloric budget"—and its relationship to cancer is of great interest to him. Nelson notes that caloric intake drops among the elderly, while their cancer rates rise. It may well be that taking in fewer calories—especially of food of little to no nutritional value—leaves elders deprived of nutrients they need to stave off cancer, he says.

The thirst for nutritional knowledge is by no means limited to physicians and wellness professionals. A poll of attendees of A Women's Journey, an annual women's health symposium sponsored by Hopkins Medicine, showed a huge demand for more seminars devoted to the nuances of nutrition, and faculty speakers who could make sense of the flood of dietary data being unleashed on the public. In response, the Fall 2009 A Woman's Journey featured numerous talks with a nutritional component, including three seminars—led by the aforementioned Nelson, Mullin, and nutritionist Lynda McIntyre—that, like a well-balanced meal, triangulated how different research approaches are translating into smarter ways to eat for health. For Gerard Mullin, nutrition and health have always been intertwined. What's different now is the scientific rigor being applied to the field.

"My mom had the first health food store in northern New Jersey. I've cooked since I was 10," says Mullin. *"I was raised on food as medicine, and I'm glad the science has really borne out and supported what many of us were raised to believe since we were yay high."* Mullin refers to himself as an integrative gastroenterologist, the adjective referring to physicians who use complementary modalities including stress management and nutrition in their clinical practices. In both interviews and talks, Mullin lays out a compelling explanation for the mind/body connection to the gut, and how different foods, spices, and herbs can promote better digestive health, especially in the 90 million Americans suffering from digestive diseases. He focuses on the common negative feedback loop affecting the "cephalic" phase of digestion—the gastric and

saliva secretions that occur when appetite is stimulated but before eating actually begins. Sleep deprivation, emotional upset, poor eating habits—all can lead to an impaired cephalic phase. It's the stomach's equivalent of not being in the mood, and the response is somewhat the same. Diminished blood flow impairs function: In this case the gut doesn't absorb nutrients. All that unabsorbed food can make us miserable (i.e., everything from diarrhea to gas, bloating, and beyond). That jacks up stress levels, makes eating even more undesirable, and before you know it you've worked yourself into a case of irritable bowel syndrome or worse.

While drugs can treat symptoms, Mullin says breaking the cycle is both a mental and physical process. Taking the time to cook can in itself enhance that first cephalic phase—everything from the meditative act of chopping to inhaling rich aromas can be relaxing—while choosing certain foods such as peppermint leaves and ground flax may reduce gut spasms.

1 in 3 people aged 65+ are at risk of malnutrition on admission to hospital

According to British Medical Journal studies, Mullin says, *"Peppermint works better than most IBS drugs. It works on relaxing calcium channel blockers. Sometimes it can make your gut so relaxed, right between the gut and esophagus, that you get some burping or heartburn, so you have to be careful how much you use. More isn't always better."*

At Hopkins, Mullin has worked to improve both nutrition and timely access to food given to Johns Hopkins Hospital inpatients. *"In a hospital setting, anywhere from 33% to 55% of people are malnourished,"* he notes. With study funding from Department of

Medicine Chief Mike Weisfeldt, says Mullin, "we proved that if you feed people earlier (following admission), their hospital stay is shorter and outcome is much better. It is common sense, but we had to show the evidence. And it's reawakened a whole discussion" about improving gut health through diet. Mullin notes that many common kitchen staples can be very effective for preventing and relieving gut-related maladies. *"Caraway has been well-studied,"* Mullin says. *"Its oil is a treatment for gastroparesis, so for those with slow motility and problems with their upper GI tract, caraway can promote motility. Fennel, ginger, dill, cumin...all these things can help you on an everyday basis."*

From both a taste and nutrient viewpoint, fresh is generally better than dried, though dried is better than nothing. As for amounts, most research suggests moderation as a key, the idea being that it's the continuous, sustainable addition of herbs and other nutrients that enhance flavor and long-term gut health. Do not skip meals, eating regularly and including herbs and spices, fruit and vegetables, and fish is truly necessary to optimum health especially in our young and elderly.

22% of people aged 60+ **skipped meals** to cut back on **food costs**

Equally important is what foods to avoid. Improving that cephalic response will be pretty much a waste if the gut is being overdosed with junk. Mullin cites studies noting that, while the average American consumes 100 grams of fructose a day—everything from "soda to ketchup to grapes"—the body can only tolerate about 50 grams. The overload acts as an IBS and gas trigger. *"The first thing we do is say, 'Look, if you want to get better, you have to find a way to eliminate some of these sugars."* He says.

Mullin aims his last culinary salvo at inflammation. Many scientists believe that certain aspects of lifestyle—notably what we eat—can create a chronic inflammatory state within cells, tissues, and organs. In short, the immune system is in constant attack mode, which may have deleterious effects on health. *"We know that many conditions in the gut are mediated through inflammation. We're appreciating that now more than ever,"* he says, pointing to recent research links. *"How do you help make yourself better? Again, it's a food as medicine approach. There are (anti-inflammatory) studies about blueberries and blackberries out there (see "Allies in the Pantry.")*

Bill Nelson's interest in food literally comes down to a flip of the wrist. No, not as a chef, but rather a scientist fascinated by how foods—notably meats—are altered by the way they're cooked. Using World Health Organization data, Nelson concluded that some 35% of cancers probably include a dietary element, with inflammation—which could also have dietary factors—playing a role in perhaps another 30% of cases. A highly respected molecular biologist and cancer clinician—he's principal investigator for one of the National Cancer Institute's Specialized Program of Research Excellence (SPORE) initiatives—Nelson has taken a microscopic interest in the interplay of diet and prostate cancer. He notes that not only do Asian men have far less prostate cancer than their American counterparts, they appear far less prone to inflammation. When comparing autopsies of non-cancerous prostates of men who live in America versus those in Asia, *"Every prostate removed here showed signs of inflammation, while the Asian prostates were pristine."* Curiously, the longer Asian men are in America, the more likely they are to develop prostate cancer. *"If they're here 25 years or more, their rate becomes half that of Caucasians, and if their kids are born here, their risk is the same as Caucasians. There must be something in the lifestyle risks that we can reduce."* While Asians tend to eat far more fish and far less meat and fowl than Americans, Nelson says that might not tell the whole story. The problem may lie in how we heat our meats. *"Heat changes a huge amount of the components in food,"* says Nelson, focusing on two particular carcinogens that can be created by cooking. The first, called heterocyclic amines, are formed by the heat-catalyzed interplay between creatinine (found in the muscle of meats and fish) and amino acids.

One heterocyclic amine called "PhIP" is extremely nasty: When given to rats in doses comparable to those consumed by humans, the male rats rapidly developed prostate and colon cancer, while the female rats developed colon and breast cancer.

"For us, that was fascinating," recalled Nelson. *"We just said, 'Holy cow! It is incredible that something you could eat could do that."*

37%
of people aged
70+ who have recently moved into care homes are at risk of
malnutrition

Not only can the amount and duration of heat increase these dangerous amines (i.e., well-done appears worse for you than medium or medium rare), but so can cooking technique. *"You can take burger patties, put them on the same skillet, control for temperature and time, but in one case you flip them only once, in the middle of cooking, while the other you flip every 30 seconds."* The burgers only flipped once *"make a ton of amines,"* notes Nelson. *"So did sausages cooked as links versus patties."* The links, in Nelson's opinion, act *"as closed reaction vessels."* Nelson's own research uncovered that in many cases the liver can't metabolize all these "charred" meat carcinogens, and passes them through to the prostate, where people with a particular DNA mutation may be at much higher risk for developing cancer.

Nelson also points out that the fat dripping along a deep grilled steak might taste delicious, but it's potentially deadly. The culprit, which also escapes from the fat in chicken skin, is something called polycyclic aromatic hydrocarbon carcinogens. To put some numbers to the science, Nelson says the amount of these carcinogens consumed daily by the average American *"equals ingesting half a pack of cigarette smoke a day."*

My suggestion: **If you're going to eat meat, and I am, then stick to lower-fat cuts, take the skin off of chicken before cooking, and look at alternatives such as broiling or, in the case of fish, poaching the filet. Remember too that fat in the diet is important, but it is the right fats – like olive oil or the fats that are found in fish that we need – not a ton of beef or poultry fats.**

Nelson believes that both the public and industry are ready to hear his message. In meetings with executives at a large grocery store, Nelson discovered that 16% of the chain's sales came from pre-cooked foods and meals that busy customers quickly reheated at home. The executives had quite an appetite for Nelson's food prep science. Not only would such techniques improve food safety, but long term, the executives saw such preparatory expertise as potentially marketable to health-conscious consumers. *"I'm tantalized by the way we could affect broad-based cooking practices,"* he says *"We're at the dawn of an era of figuring this out."*

Figuring out how to translate serious science into tasty, healthy snacks and meals is where nutritionist Lynda McIntyre excels. A registered dietitian with a specialty counseling cancer patients at both the Kimmel Cancer Center at Hopkins and the Sibley Hospital Center for Breast Health in Washington D.C., McIntyre took A Woman's Journey attendees on a virtual tour of the supermarket.

Along the way, she busted some myths regarding what it is about food that links it to perhaps the majority of cancer cases.

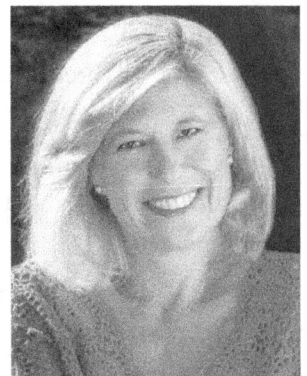

"A lot of times people think I'm talking about pesticides or additives in food, when in fact I'm not," she says. *"Less than 2% percent of all cancers can be directly related to what the additives are in food. Up to 60 percent can be related to what we're not eating."*

<u>Read that quote again</u> – I know that we are all concerned about pesticides in our food, as we should be, but we need to be at least equally concerned about what **we are and are not eating!** As in enough fruits and vegetables. A familiar message, yes, but McIntyre gives it a twist, suggesting shoppers take a colorful approach to solving their qualms about which produce has the greatest overall benefits. You have heard me say it and now this doctor stresses it too, *"Eat the rainbow. The brighter the food, the richer the color, the higher its anti-oxidant count,"* counsels McIntyre, who also served on a statewide council that developed cancer prevention strategies for Maryland. For McIntyre and other savvy nutritionists, the state of food science has allowed them to fine-tune their message and take some of the confusion out of the game. Take fresh versus frozen produce. McIntyre says both are effective…

"Fresh is always best when it is in season," says McIntyre, since fresh produce retains top flavor and nutritional value. However, McIntyre notes that many fresh foods have relatively short seasons. As an alternative, from a nutritional viewpoint, *"frozen can be just as nutritious because it's picked at the peak of ripeness, and frozen to keep the nutritional content intact."*

Then there's eating whole foods versus taking supplements, a source of huge debate. The prevailing sentiment among many researchers is that supplementation can bring someone deficient in a given nutrient up to a supportive

93% 🍴

of malnourished

older people are in the

community.

baseline, but people already at solid baseline levels may not benefit from additional dosing.

"In some cases, single supplementation of antioxidants can increase the risk of certain diseases," says McIntyre. *"For example, vitamin E and heart disease. Another example is that single supplementation of vitamin A can increase bone fractures in women. And in smokers who took beta-carotene, we saw an increase in lung cancer. The studies show it is the whole foods (and how they work together synergistically) that provides the most protective effect to the body."*

Knowing how to combine those foods can increase the body's ability to absorb their nutrients. McIntyre says putting broccoli (sulforaphane) and tomatoes (lycopene) together *"increases their tumor protective ability."* Similarly, carrots and avocado are a nice dynamic duo because beta-carotene is better absorbed in the presence of a fat (short on avocados? Try olive oil). Apples and blueberries, even spinach and strawberries (*"It's a strange combination, but delicious,"* insists McIntyre) all make for nutrient-dense dynamic duos.

    So, bottom line, what I want, and need, for you to understand is this; as for the thinking that healthy eating and drinking is restrictive, forget it. Nearly every family of food and beverage that I have researched—be it nut, fruit, spice, fish, grain, beans, chocolate, wine, beer or coffee, has some and very often many, members in it filled with high nutritional content, when we consume them in moderation. On every conceivable front, from the molecular level to the kitchen table, research is unlocking the power of certain foods and drinks to keep us in fighting shape. Since none of us has a "foodprint" yet—a DNA or some other molecular roadmap that will tell us why Sally's system can absorb beta-carotene from carrots, while Sue's can only assimilate that same beta-carotene from sweet potatoes—for now, eating a well-rounded, well-informed diet containing moderate amounts of a wide varieties of fresh foods and drinks, is all about playing the odds. And there's nothing better than improving your chances of beating the house.

So, the next time that someone tries to tell you that you shouldn't be eating that freshly roasted corn on the cob, – just tell them that they shouldn't worry, you are just working on improving your health!

Chapter 9: The Health Benefits of Corn

The health benefits of corn include controlling diabetes, prevention of heart ailments, lowering hypertension and prevention of neural-tube defects at birth. Corn or maize is one of the most popular cereals in the world and forms the staple food in many countries, including the United States and many African countries.

The kernels of corn are what hold the majority of corn's nutrients, and are the most commonly consumed parts of the vegetable. The kernels can come in multiple colors, depending on where the corn is grown and what species or variety they happen to be. Another genetic variant, called sweetcorn, has more sugar and less starch in the nutritive material.

Corn not only provides the necessary calories for healthy, daily metabolism, but is also a rich source of vitamin A, vitamin B, vitamin E, and many minerals. Its high fiber content ensures that it plays a significant role in the prevention of digestive ailments like constipation and hemorrhoids as well as colorectal cancer. The antioxidants present in corn also act as anti-carcinogenic agents and prevent Alzheimer's disease.

Corn provides many health benefits due to the presence of quality nutrients within. Besides being a delicious addition to any meal, it is also rich in phytochemicals, and it provides protection against a number of chronic diseases. Some of the well-researched and widespread health benefits of corn are listed below.

- **Rich source of calories:** Corn is a rich source of calories and is a staple among dietary habits in many populations. The calorific content of corn is 342 calories per 100 grams, which is among the highest for cereals. It is why corn is often turned to for quick weight gain, and combined with the ease and flexibility of growing conditions for corn, the high calorie content makes it vital for the survival of dozens of agricultural-based nations.

- **Reduces risk of hemorrhoids and colorectal cancer:** The fiber content of one cup of corn amounts to 18.4% of the daily recommended amount. This aids in alleviating digestive problems such as constipation and hemorrhoids, as well as lowering the risk of colon cancer due to corn being a whole-grain. Fiber has long been promoted as a way to reduce colon risk, but insufficient and conflicting data exists for fiber's relationship with preventing cancer, although whole-grain consumption, on the whole, has been proven to reduce that risk. Fiber helps to bulk up bowel movements, which stimulates peristaltic motion and even stimulates the production of gastric juice and bile. It can also add bulk to overly loose stools, which can slow reduce the chances of Irritable Bowel Syndrome (IBS) and diarrhea.

- **Rich source of vitamins:** Corn is rich in vitamin B constituents, especially Thiamin and Niacin. Thiamin is essential for maintaining nerve health and cognitive function. Niacin deficiency leads to Pellagra; a disease characterized by diarrhea, dementia and dermatitis that is commonly observed in malnourished individuals. Corn is also a good source of Pantothenic acid, which is an essential vitamin for carbohydrate, protein, and lipid metabolism in the body. Deficiency of folic acid in pregnant women can lead to the birth of underweight infants and may also result in neural tube defects in newborns. Corn provides a large percentage of the daily folate requirement, while the kernels of corn are rich in vitamin E, a natural antioxidant that is essential for growth and protection of the body from illness and disease.

- **Provides necessary minerals:** Corn contains abundant minerals which positively benefit the bodies in a number of ways. phosphorous, along with magnesium, manganese, zinc, iron and copper are found in all varieties of corn. It also contains trace minerals like selenium, which are difficult to find in most normal diets. Phosphorous is essential for regulating normal growth, bone health and optimal kidney functioning. Magnesium is necessary for maintaining a normal heart rate and for increasing bone strength.

- **Antioxidant properties:** According to studies carried out at Cornell University, corn is a rich source of antioxidants which fight cancer-causing free radicals. In fact, unlike many other foods, cooking actually increases the amount of usable antioxidants in sweet corn. Corn is a rich source of a phenolic compound called ferulic acid, an anti-carcinogenic agent that has been shown to be effective in fighting the tumors which lead to breast cancer as well as liver cancer. Anthocyanins, found in purple corn, also act as scavengers and eliminators of cancer-causing free radicals. Antioxidants have been shown to reduce many of the most dangerous forms of cancer because of their ability to induce apoptosis in cancerous cells, while leaving healthy cells unaffected. This is particularly relevant when phytochemicals are the source of the antioxidants, which is another type of chemical found in high volumes in corn.

- **Protecting Your Heart:** According to researchers, corn oil has been shown to have an anti-atherogenic effect on cholesterol levels, thus reducing the risk of various cardiovascular diseases. Corn oil, particularly, is the best way to increase heart health, and this is derived from the fact that corn is close to an optimal fatty acid combination. This allows omega-3 fatty acids to strip away the damaging "bad" cholesterol and replace them at the binding sites. This will reduce the chances of arteries becoming clogged, will reduce blood pressure, and decrease the change of heart attack and stroke.
- **Prevents Anemia:** Corn helps to prevent anemia caused by deficiency of these vitamins. Corn also has a significant level of iron, which is one of the essential minerals needed to form new red blood cells; a deficiency in iron is one of the main cause of anemia as well.
- **Lowers LDL Cholesterol:** According to the Journal of Nutritional Biochemistry, consumption of corn husk oil lowers plasma LDL cholesterol by reducing cholesterol absorption in the body. As mentioned earlier, this reduction of LDL cholesterol does not mean a reduction in HDL cholesterol, which is considered "good cholesterol" and can have a variety of beneficial effects on the body, including the reduction of heart disease, prevention of atherosclerosis, and a general scavenger of free radicals throughout the body.
- **Vitamin-A Content:** Yellow corn is a rich source of beta-carotene, which forms vitamin A in the body and is essential for the maintenance of good vision and skin. Beta-carotene is a great source of vitamin-A because it is converted within the body, but only in the amounts that the body requires. Vitamin-A can be toxic if too much is consumed, so deriving vitamin-A through beta-carotene transformation is ideal.

Vitamin-A will also benefit the health of skin and mucus membranes, as well as boosting the immune system.

- The amount of beta-carotene in the body that is not converted into vitamin-A acts as a very strong antioxidant, like all carotenoids, and can combat terrible diseases like cancer and heart disease. That being said, smokers need to be careful about their beta-carotene content, because smokers with high beta-carotene levels are more likely to contract lung cancer, while non-smokers with high beta-carotene content are less likely to contract lung cancer.

- **Controls diabetes and hypertension:** In recent decades, the world has seemed to suffer from an epidemic of diabetes. Although the exact mechanism for this cannot be pinpointed, it is generally assumed to relate to nutrition. Eating more organic fruits and vegetables, like corn, has been thought to be a return to an older style of diet, and it has been linked to reduced signs of diabetes. Studies have shown that the consumption of corn kernels assists in the management of non-insulin dependent diabetes mellitus (NIDDM) and is effective against hypertension due to the presence of phenolic phytochemicals in whole corn. Phytochemicals can regulate the absorption and release of insulin in the body, which can reduce the chance of spikes and drops for diabetic patients and help them maintain a more normal lifestyle.

- **Cosmetic benefits:** Corn starch is used in the manufacturing of many cosmetic products and may also be applied topically to soothe skin rashes and irritation. Corn products can be used to replace carcinogenic petroleum products which are major components of many cosmetic preparations. Many of the traditional skin creams contain petroleum jelly as a base material, which can often block pores and make skin conditions even worse.

A Few Words of Warning: Corn does contain large amounts of fatty acid, so for people who are already at high risk for heart disease, excess corn or corn oil can dangerously exacerbate those conditions and risks. Also, corn is frequently turned into high fructose corn syrup, which is extracted from corn to use as a cheap sweetener. It is worse than table sugar and is a cause of obesity, as well as having a negative impact on your blood sugar levels. It is found in many artificially sweetened foods and syrups, so avoid these if you want to only get the positive benefits of corn.

Corn is a rich source of many essential nutrients and fiber. A meal rich in corn can go a long way in protecting against many diseases and ailments. So start shucking!

Conclusion

I have used this exact same conclusion is several of my book and this one will be no different! While I could bow to convention and follow the "rules" of proper book layout and publishing, those that demand that in the conclusion I sum up all of the preceding chapters and answer any questions that may still remain in the minds of my readers, I would rather not.

Frankly I just don't want to do that. So, since I have never much been one for following all the "rules," I think I'll just approach this conclusion the way I want.

You see, I absolutely do not want to answer all of your questions with this book. In fact, I think that all of those so called, "all you need to know" books are ridiculous!

What I want to achieve with this work, what hope I have achieved is that I provided you with enough solid, scientific information and historical fact, that you are encouraged to start asking more questions about everything you consume; their history, their impact on mankind, and their possible impact on your health. I hope you do some additional research of your own!

As for how I would sum up this book? Let me simply paraphrase something I have said many times…

Too much of a good thing is not a good thing! Ridiculously increased corn consumption over time will not lead to better health but could, and usually will, in fact, ruin your health.

Moderation is the key word here!

For more information on health, nutrition, gardening, phytonutrition, antioxidants and loads more please visit my website and while you are there go ahead and subscribe to my phytonutrient blog – its free but the information is priceless!

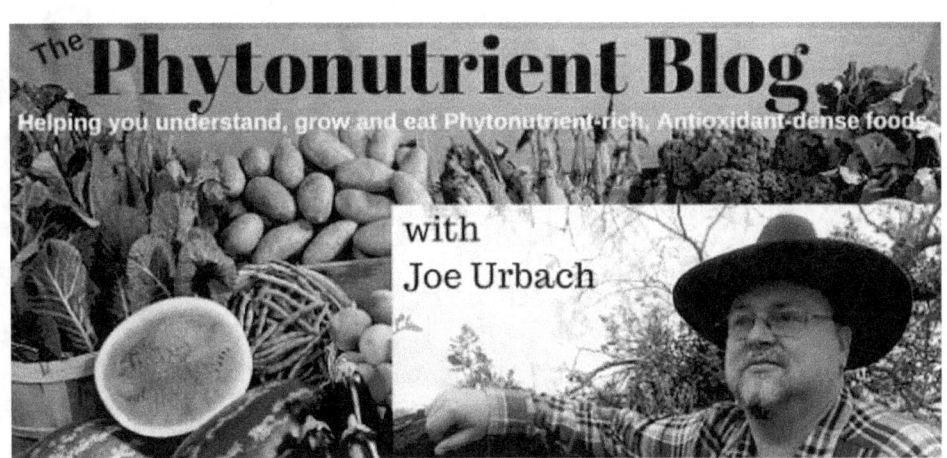

www.GardeningAustin.com/blog

For the highest quality, hand sourced, Organic, NON-GMO seeds for you garden visit:

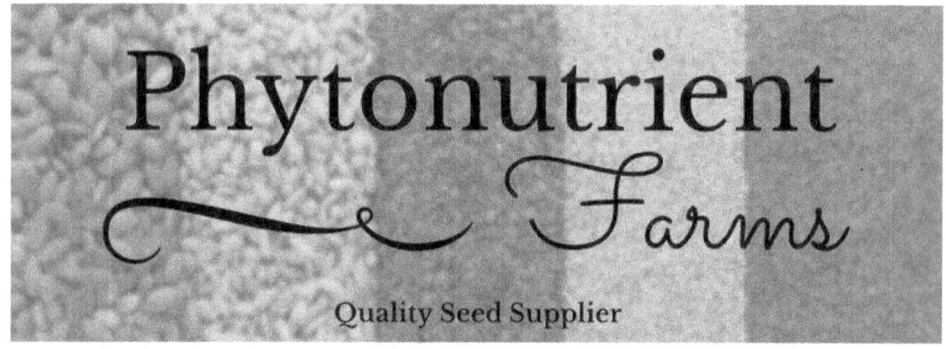

www.phytonutrientfarms.com

I will leave you with just a few more bits of graphical information to consider. If nothing I have written in this book has got you thinking than maybe one of these will:

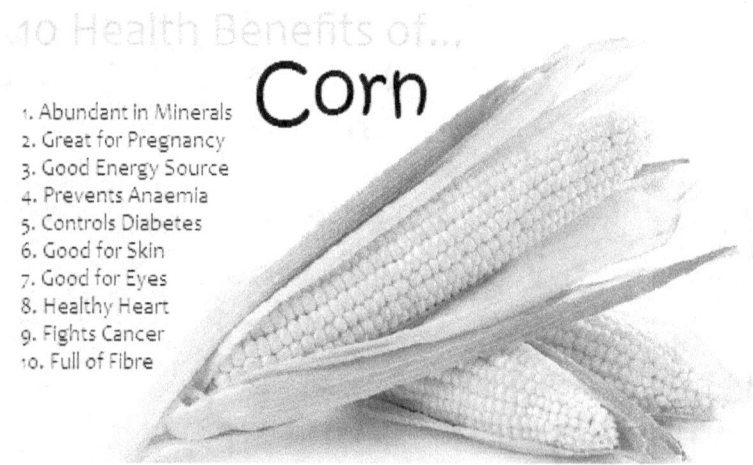

10 Health Benefits of...

Corn

1. Abundant in Minerals
2. Great for Pregnancy
3. Good Energy Source
4. Prevents Anaemia
5. Controls Diabetes
6. Good for Skin
7. Good for Eyes
8. Healthy Heart
9. Fights Cancer
10. Full of Fibre

The Corny Truth About
HIGH FRUCTOSE CORN SYRUP

Top 10 Foods with the Highest Quantity of HFCS:

1) Yogurt	6) Boxed Mac n Cheese
2) Breads	7) Salad Dressing
3) Frozen Pizza	8) Tomato-Based Sauces
4) Cereal Bars	9) Apple Sauce
5) Cocktail Peanuts	10) Canned Fruit

*High Fructose Corn Syrup has been linked directly to obesity, diabetes and metabolic dysfunction

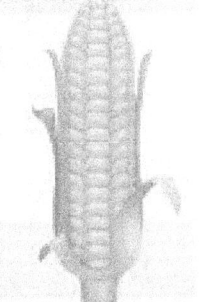

HEALTH BENEFITS OF CORN

ESSENTIAL DURING PREGNANCY

CONTROLS CHOLESTEROL

SKIN CARE

PREVENTS ANEMIA

A POWER HOUSE OF MINERALS

IMPROVES DIGESTION

NUTRITION FACTS
SWEET CORN

SWEET CORN, WHITE
AMOUNT PER 100 GRAMS
CALORIES 86
OR LOWER DEPENDING ON YOUR CALORIE NEEDS.

TOTAL CARBOHYDRATE 19 G	6%	
DIETARY FIBER	2.7 G	10%
SUGAR	3.2 G	
PROTEIN	3.2 G 6%	
VITAMIN A	0.0%	
VITAMIN C	11%	
CALCIUM	0%	
IRON	2%	
VITAMIN B-6	5%	
VITAMIN B-12	0%	
MAGNESIUM	9%	

SATURATED FAT	0.2 G
POLYUNSATURATED FAT	0.6 G
MONOUNSATURATED FAT	0.3 G
CHOLESTEROL 0 MG	0%
SODIUM 15 MG	0%
POTASSIUM 270 MG	0%7

Pros

1. Good Source of Antioxidants
Carotenoid antioxidants, the kind most abundant in corn kernels, are known to support the immune system and defend the eyes and skin against oxidative stress.

2. High in Fiber
Like all vegetables and whole plant foods, corn is a food that provides a nice dose of filling fiber, with about 4.5 grams of fiber per cup of kernels. It has a high ratio of insoluble-to-soluble fiber, which means it has various beneficial effects on the digestive system.

3. Slowly Digested Source of Carbohydrates
Corn is high in starch, which is a type of complex carbohydrate that supports steady energy levels. Unlike refined carbohydrates, which zap us of energy and aren't filling for long, foods high in starch and fiber are beneficial for controlling blood sugar levels because the fiber slows down the rate at which glucose (sugar) is released into the bloodstream.

4. Naturally Gluten-Free
Although corn is usually grouped together with other grains and used in similar ways, it's actually not a "grain" and doesn't contain any gluten.

Cons

1. When It's Genetically Modified
Corn is the No. 1 grown crop in the Unites States and currently the second most genetically modified ingredient in the world (second to soy). About 88 percent of all corn grown in the U.S. each year is genetically modified.

2. When It's Used to Make High Fructose Corn Syrup
Despite what manufacturers might make it seem like, high fructose corn syrup isn't natural and is the furthest thing from being healthy.

3. When It's Found in Other Forms of Processed Foods
GMO corn is used to make dozens of different ingredients added to packaged, processed foods. Before you buy any food product, always read the entire food label to make sure the product is safe and generally free from anything you can't pronounce.

4. If You Have a Sensitive Digestive System
Even though corn is gluten-free and technically not a grain, it's possible for corn to still aggravate your digestive system and cause stomachaches, especially if you suffer from other common food allergies, sensitivities to FODMAP foods, IBS or leaky gut syndrome.

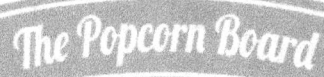

NUTRITIONAL
INFORMATION

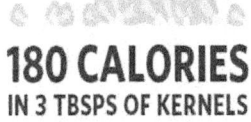

180 CALORIES
IN 3 TBSPS OF KERNELS

+

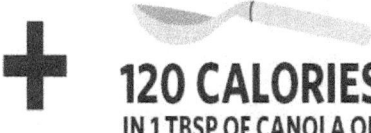

120 CALORIES*
IN 1 TBSP OF CANOLA OIL

35 CALORIES
IN 1 CUP OF
OIL-POPPED POPCORN

210 CALORIES
IN 6 CUPS OF POPCORN

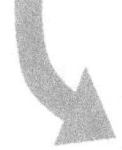

2 SERVINGS 7 GRAMS
OF GRAINS OF FIBER

*Some oil remains in the popper

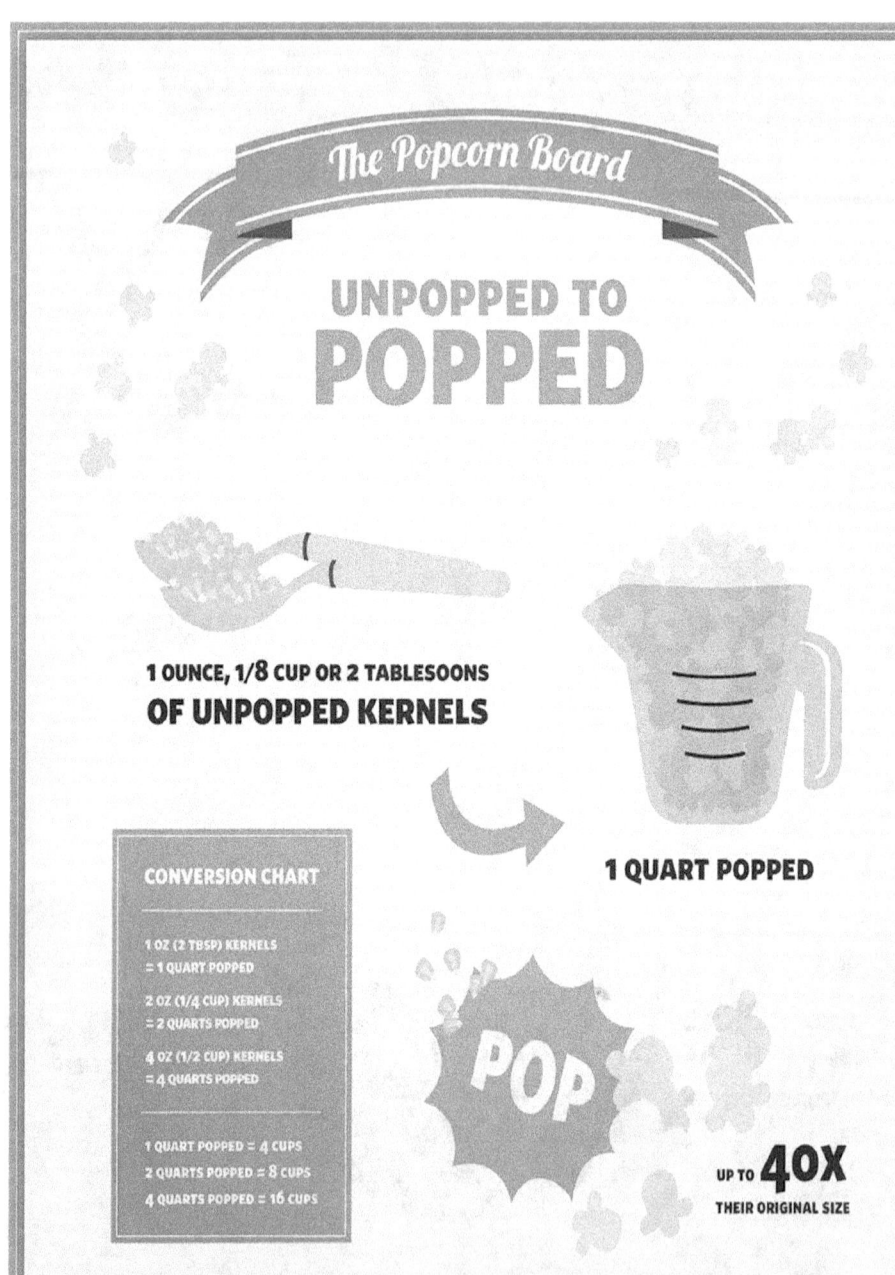

The Popcorn Board

UNPOPPED TO
POPPED

**1 OUNCE, 1/8 CUP OR 2 TABLESOONS
OF UNPOPPED KERNELS**

1 QUART POPPED

CONVERSION CHART

1 OZ (2 TBSP) KERNELS
= 1 QUART POPPED

2 OZ (1/4 CUP) KERNELS
= 2 QUARTS POPPED

4 OZ (1/2 CUP) KERNELS
= 4 QUARTS POPPED

1 QUART POPPED = 4 CUPS
2 QUARTS POPPED = 8 CUPS
4 QUARTS POPPED = 16 CUPS

POP

UP TO **40X**
THEIR ORIGINAL SIZE

The Popcorn Board

INDUSTRY
FACTS

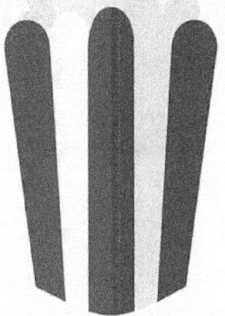

13.5%
MOISTURE

IDEAL FOR POPABILITY

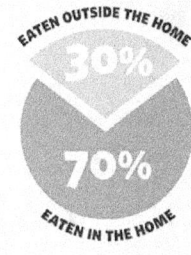

EATEN OUTSIDE THE HOME

30%

70%

EATEN IN THE HOME

9 MAJOR POPCORN PRODUCING STATES

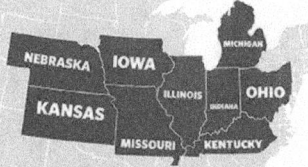

NEBRASKA IOWA MICHIGAN
ILLINOIS INDIANA OHIO
KANSAS
MISSOURI KENTUCKY

51
QUARTS
CONSUMED

/ PER PERSON
ANNUALLY

AMERICANS CONSUME
16 BILLION
QUARTS OF POPCORN ANNUALLY

4 MAIN TYPES
OF CORN

SWEET   **FIELD**

FLINT   **POPCORN**

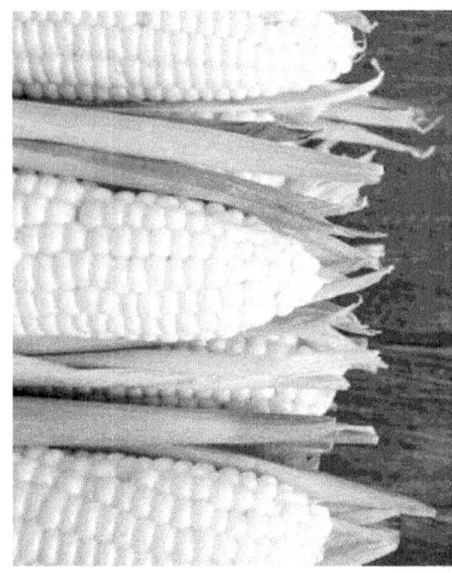

The Bottom Line on Corn

Organic, non-GMO corn can be a part of an otherwise balanced and healthy diet, but the same can't be said for GMO corn and processed corn-derivative ingredients.

How can you be sure you're not consuming GMO corn? Without proper labeling, avoiding any ingredient made with GMO corn can be very hard, so the key is to eat real whole foods and avoid those that come in packages as much as possible.

The Great
Corn Debate

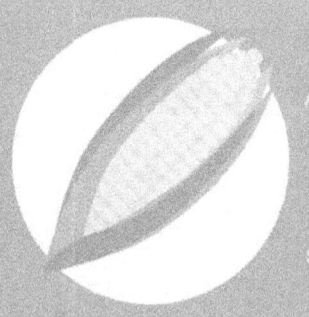

Corn was first domesticated over 8,000 years ago and is a traditional food for Native Americans. It's also been a staple ingredient in South, Central and North American for thousands of years.

The nutritional value of corn has helped support growing populations, especially living in impoverished areas, for many years.

Real, traditional corn is grown throughout the warm summer months on stalks of "ears" that come in far more colors than the standard bright yellow; corn can be found in different varieties, including red, pink, black, purple, multicolored and blue.

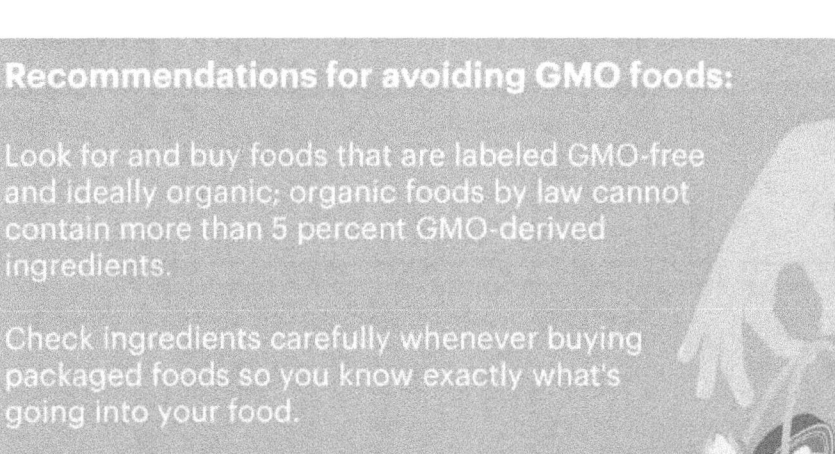

Recommendations for avoiding GMO foods:

Look for and buy foods that are labeled GMO-free and ideally organic; organic foods by law cannot contain more than 5 percent GMO-derived ingredients.

Check ingredients carefully whenever buying packaged foods so you know exactly what's going into your food.

Avoid all foods with corn oil (or other refined vegetable oils like canola and safflower that are also likely GMO).

Avoid foods made with high fructose corn syrup.

Shop at your local farmers market and ask about the quality of the corn.

Considering growing your own corn (using non-GMO seeds!) so you know you're eating the freshest and highest quality you can.

To find more books by this author visit...

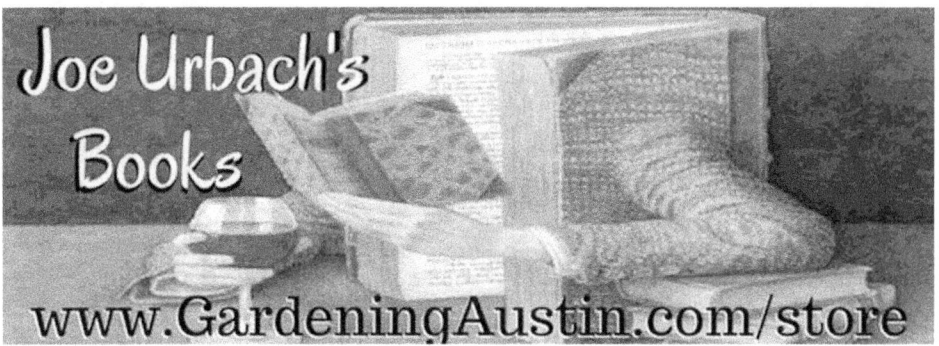

Joe Urbach's Books

www.GardeningAustin.com/store

www.ingramcontent.com/pod-product-compliance
Lightning Source LLC
Chambersburg PA
CBHW072144280526
45788CB00002B/775